Clinical Methods in
CARDIOLOGY

Clinical Methods in
CARDIOLOGY

RS Sharma

MD Medicine DM Cardiology (AIIMS, New Delhi) FICP

Senior Consultant and In-Charge
Department of Cardiology
Government Medical College
Jabalpur, Madhya Pradesh, India

Foreword
DP Lokwani

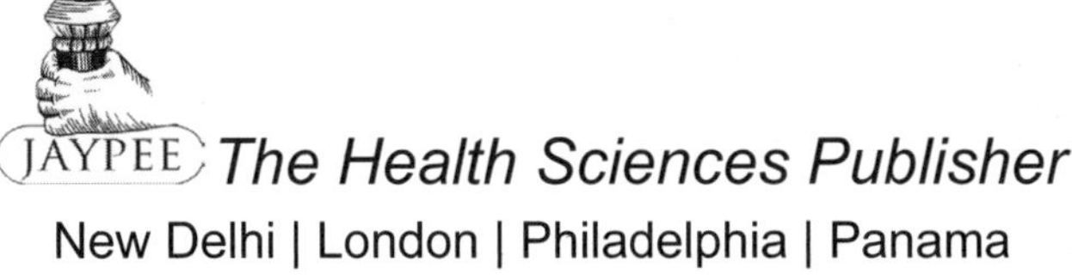

The Health Sciences Publisher
New Delhi | London | Philadelphia | Panama

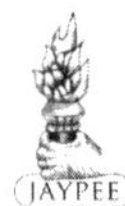 **Jaypee Brothers Medical Publishers (P) Ltd**

Headquarters

Jaypee Brothers Medical Publishers (P) Ltd
4838/24, Ansari Road, Daryaganj
New Delhi 110 002, India
Phone: +91-11-43574357
Fax: +91-11-43574314
Email: jaypee@jaypeebrothers.com

Overseas Offices

J.P. Medical Ltd
83, Victoria Street, London
SW1H 0HW (UK)
Phone: +44 20 3170 8910
Fax: +44 (0) 20 3008 6180
Email: info@jpmedpub.com

Jaypee Medical Inc
The Bourse
111 South Independence Mall East
Suite 835, Philadelphia, PA 19106, USA
Phone: +1 267-519-9789
Email: jpmed.us@gmail.com

Jaypee Brothers Medical Publishers (P) Ltd
Bhotahity, Kathmandu, Nepal
Phone: +977-9741283608
Email: kathmandu@jaypeebrothers.com

Jaypee-Highlights Medical Publishers Inc.
City of Knowledge, Bld. 237, Clayton
Panama City, Panama
Phone: +1 507-301-0496
Fax: +1 507-301-0499
Email: cservice@jphmedical.com

Jaypee Brothers Medical Publishers (P) Ltd
17/1-B Babar Road, Block-B, Shaymali
Mohammadpur, Dhaka-1207
Bangladesh
Mobile: +08801912003485
Email: jaypeedhaka@gmail.com

Website: www.jaypeebrothers.com
Website: www.jaypeedigital.com

Inquiries for bulk sales may be solicited at: jaypee@jaypeebrothers.com

Clinical Methods in Cardiology

First Edition: **2015**

ISBN 978-93-5152-665-0

Printed at Rajkamal Electric Press, Plot No. 2, Phase-IV, Kundli, Haryana.

Dedicated to

The invisible, but omnipresent divinity
My parents, Shri DD Sharma and Mrs Santosh Sharma
My wife, Dr Archana Sharma
My twin daughters – Dr Supriya Sharma and Dr Shilpa Sharma
My son, Siddhartha Sharma (Aspiring Cardiothoracic Surgeon)
and
My teachers, students and all my patients ...!

FOREWORD

The expert knowledge regarding clinical examination in cardiology shall be very useful and important for the undergraduate and postgraduate students, and those pursuing superspecialization in cardiology. The author has a sound academic background and this book reflects his 30 years of post-DM experience in field as a Senior Consultant and In-Charge in Cardiology at Government Medical College, Jabalpur, Madhya Pradesh, India. The contents list is complete and chapters have been written pretty well. The book comprises of compilation of proper history taking, clinical examination methods, physical signs and their correlation in order to arrive at a definite diagnosis. The author has also adopted an individual disease-wise approach that provides an in-depth knowledge rather than a superficial brushing up. Beautiful diagrams and photographs add to the teaching value of this most comprehensive book on clinical cardiology seen by me for a long time.

I am sure that this book will not only be useful in providing knowledge but also in stimulating innovative motivation in the field of cardiology.

DP Lokwani
Vice-Chancellor
Madhya Pradesh University of Medical Sciences
Jabalpur, Madhya Pradesh, India

PREFACE

Welcome to the fascinating and rewarding world of cardiology. This book *Clinical Methods in Cardiology* seems a little too ambitious; however, every seasoned medical teacher is aware of the fact that a 'Postgraduate Student' is actually a 'Very Good Undergraduate Student'. You cannot be a good MD, without being a very good MBBS.

I wish to point out that this is not a textbook of cardiology, nor was it meant to be. Rather, it is a Senior Cardiologist's attempt to accumulate and present in a pleasant manner all the relevant cardiology practice information in an applied form for 'Clinical Cardiology'.

I have had the opportunity to learn cardiology from my distinguished professors in 'Mecca of Cardiology' in India—the 'All India Institute of Medical Sciences, New Delhi'. Here, I learnt to look for ways to apply all the knowledge acquired in a practical sense.

Of course, I am also aware of the fact that besides accumulating knowledge, it is also essential to pass in examination with excellence; hence, I have deliberately made certain chapters of this book 'examination friendly', so as to generate more confidence in the exam-going students. These questions and answers type format definitely act as a 'mental gym' and you know the rule of exercise for muscles 'use it or lose it' this is also true for brain.

Hoping to generate among undergraduates, postgraduates and residents a genuine interest in cardiology by this small effort of mine.

RS Sharma

ACKNOWLEDGMENTS

- I acknowledge with thanks from the bottom of my heart the contribution of my parents, without whom I would not have been in this great world. Father especially for grooming my personality and mother for providing me an ideal stable platform called 'home'.
- My lovely wife, my twin daughters (now both doctors), and a vibrant teenaged son aspiring to be Cardiothoracic Surgeon, who contributed by allowing me to complete this book at the 'expense of their time'. Without them, the book could have been completed much earlier but then life would not have been so much fun and worth living.
- All my teachers who taught me 'how to learn yourself'.
- All my patients who actually are the real teachers of this fascinating subject.
- Finally, the typist who has done the herculean task of deciphering my handwriting and typing it too.

CONTENTS

Chapter 1

History Taking

A detailed but not time wasting history is essential and most useful part of diagnosis making. Sometime nonverbal "Body language" gives tremendous information. Mood, distress anxiety can be seen better but may not be said.

The physician's questioning should be unhurried and nonthreatening but nonetheless thorough. Skillful interrogation, appropriate to the urgency of the situation, must be matched by thoughtful listening. Questions should not be suggestive of answer.

The patient must be encouraged to raise questions at appropriate times.

Artful history taking brings the patient and physician close together. For this reason, it is a critical factor not only in establishing the diagnosis but also in determining the outcome of subsequent therapy.

Proper communication is the lifeline of a good history. Communication is a bigger thing than history taking (Fig. 1.1).

▌ SUBCLINICAL DISEASE; ▌ ASYMPTOMATIC PATIENTS

The modern tendency for patients with no symptoms to consult physicians for routine "checkup" examinations has increased the likelihood that doctors will cause unnecessary anxiety in their patients even though the intent of such examinations is to discover latent or

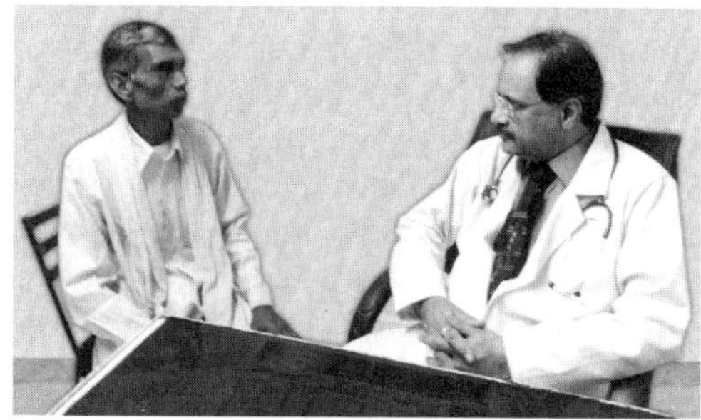

Fig. 1.1: Proper history taking establishes good communication and is valuable in diagnosis making

developing illness. Since symptoms of disease are often exaggerations of normal findings (e.g. dyspnea, fatigue), the borderline between normality and disease is often difficult to define. The problem becomes greater as the patient becomes older because the range of normality widens with advancing years. Some patients deny the existence of symptoms, fearing to be told that they are ill and may die; and some may exaggerate symptoms, if being ill seems to have usefulness as a weapon or problem-solving device. Decreasing activity, failing memory, and wishful thinking may lead people to defer seeking advice until disease is far-advanced. Persons with no complaints are technically not "patients", and a distinction should be maintained between conditions discovered during routine examinations and the diseases of patients with true symptoms. Experience in dealing with clinical and laboratory information

History taking is not only asking questions but is a well-practiced conversation...

obtained from checkup examinations is relatively small, and physicians tend to forget that under such circumstances they are dealing with a pre-symptomatic phase of disease. The physician should avoid unnecessary and prolonged personal talks or jokes with patients, as this is likely to reduce the "higher image" of doctor in whom patent usually finds solace. A respectful distance should be maintained in author's opinion. Ideally, a room free of noises is preferred.

The difficulty of interpreting a symptom, which may also be a normal physiologic response, is perhaps most strikingly demonstrated in the case of the cardinal symptom of heart disease—dyspnea, or shortness of breath. Shortness of breath on exertion is a normal phenomenon. In most cases, exercise performance is limited by shortness of breath rather than by fatigue, chest pain, leg pain, dizziness, or syncope. Dyspnea on progressively less severe exertion is also a normal accompaniment of the common modern combination of' a sedentary life, increasing weight, and increasing age. The insidious onset of shortness of breath on exertion—a characteristic of heart disease is thus more difficult to assess than some obviously abnormal symptom like hemoptysis or severe chest pain.

The history is crucial to make a diagnosis. Heart disease commonly occurs without abnormal physical findings; for example, examination is often normal in intermittent arrhythmias between episodes. Examination may confirm a cardiac or peripheral vascular diagnosis, e.g. when examining a patient with a murmur, heart failure or an abdominal aortic aneurysm, but physical signs may be completely absent in serious disease:

- Patients with severe carotid artery disease may have no neck bruit because flow through the stenosis is too slow
- Large abdominal aortic aneurysms can be impalpable in the obese
- Patients with extensive deep vein thrombosis often appear to have normal legs.

Presenting Complaint

Establish the frequency, duration and severity of symptoms, and causative and relieving factors. Urgently attend to breathlessness, recent chest or lower limb pain. Many cardiovascular diseases are slowly progressive and the evolution of symptoms guides the timing of investigations and treatment, e.g heart valve surgery is indicated for significantly limiting symptoms and surgery for carotid artery disease is most effective soon after a cerebral event.

Cardiovascular disease presenting with 'non-cardiac' symptoms		
System	Symptom	Cause
Central nervous system	Stroke	Cerebral embolism Endocarditis Hypertension
Gastrointestinal	Jaundice Abdominal pain	Liver congestion secondary to heart failure Mesenteric embolism
Renal	Oliguria	Heart failure

Functional Impairment

Assess the impact of symptoms on the patient's functional capacity. For chest discomfort or breathlessness, establish the intensity of exercise required to induce symptoms.

- Does gentle walking or only strenuous exercise like climbing hills or stairs provoke symptoms?
- Can patients keep up when walking with their partners or friends of the same age?
- What is the extent of domestic, e.g. cooking, cleaning, shopping; social, e.g. mobility, hobbies, sport, and occupational disability?

Light-headedness and syncope may impair confidence, raise fear of physical injury, and have significant implications for patients' safety when driving.

Calf leg pain on walking (intermittent claudication) from lower limb arterial disease is the most common symptom of peripheral vascular disease:

- How far can the patient walk before the pain comes on, and is this on the flat or uphill?

Past History

Ask about rheumatic fever or heart murmurs during childhood and conditions associated with heart disease, including:

- Smoking
- Hypertension
- Diabetes mellitus
- Kidney disease
- Thyrotoxicosis (atrial fibrillation)
- Alcohol intake (arrhythmias and cardiomyopathy)
- Marfan's syndrome (aortic regurgitation or aortic dissection).

In suspected infective endocarditis, ask about recent dental work and other potential causes of bacteremia, e.g. skin infections, intravenous drug use, penetrating trauma. Consider possible links between other organ system diseases and cardiovascular illness: for example, patients with renal failure or disseminated cancer and pericardial effusion; heart failure and cytotoxic drugs; radiotherapy and radiation arteritis in the affected area. Patients with chronic respiratory disease may develop right-sided heart failure (cor pulmonale) or atrial fibrillation. Connective tissue diseases such as rheumatoid arthritis are associated with Raynaud's phenomenon and pericarditis.

Drug History

Drugs may cause or aggravate symptoms such as breathlessness, chest pain, edema, palpitation or syncope. Starting thyroxine for hypothyroidism may precipitate or aggravate angina. 'Recreational' drugs such as cocaine and amphetamines can cause arrhythmias, chest pain and even myocardial infarction. Ask about over-the-counter purchases such as NSAIDs and alternative medicine and herbal remedies, as these may contain ingredients with cardiovascular actions. Beta-blockers may worsen the symptoms of intermittent claudication and any drug that lowers blood pressure tends to impair the peripheral circulation.

Genetically determined cardiovascular disorder	
Single-gene defects	
• Hypertrophic cardiomyopathy	• Muscular dystrophies
• Marfan's syndrome	• Long Q-T syndrome
• Familial hypercholesterolemia	
Polygenic inheritance	
• Ischemic heart disease	• Hyperlipidemia
• Hypertension	• Abdominal aortic aneurysm
• Type 2 diabetes mellitus	

Family History

Many cardiac disorders have a genetic component. Ask about a family history of either premature coronary artery disease in a first-degree relative (< 60 years in a female or < 55 years in a male) or sudden unexplained death at a young age, raising the possibility of a cardiomyopathy or inherited arrhythmia disorder. Patients with peripheral arterial and venous thrombosis may have inherited thrombophilia, Familial hypercholesterolemia is associated with premature cardiac and peripheral arterial disease.

Social History

Smoking is the strongest reversible risk factor for coronary artery disease and peripheral vascular disease. Take a detailed smoking history. Alcohol can induce atrial fibrillation, and alcohol excess is associated with obesity, hypertension and dilated cardiomyopathy. Excess alcohol intake with poor nutrition also predisposes to peripheral arterial and venous disease. Intravenous drug use can damage peripheral arteries and veins, most commonly causing an infected false aneurysm of the common femoral artery in the groin: a potential source for infective endocarditis.

Occupational History

Heart disease may impair physical activity and affect employment. This may be a source of anxiety and an indication for treatment. The diagnosis of heart disease has medicolegal consequences in certain occupations, such as commercial drivers and pilots. Workers exposed to occupational vibration using air-powered tools may develop 'vibration white finger', which presents with vasospasm (Raynaud's phenomenon) and neurosensory (numbness, tingling) symptoms.

▌DYSPNEA

Mechanism of Dyspnea

The unpleasant sensation of the need for increased ventilation is the best description of dyspnea. Two main varieties have been distinguished. With the first variety, the patient feels that extra work on the part of the respiratory muscles is required to achieve adequate ventilation. With the second type, the patient is aware of a feeling of smothering and feels an urgent need to take another breath; the smothering sensation is akin to that associated with breath holding. Dyspnea is a cortical sensation involving consciousness and must be distinguished from hyperpnea, or increased ventilation, which may occur without any discomfort or distress and which may be seen in unconscious patients or tachypnea which is increased rate.

Dyspnea in Heart Disease

The dyspnea of patients with heart disease that most closely resembles the dyspnea of normal exertion. Characteristically, it is directly related to the degree of exertion. The patient complains that some effort that previously did not result in awareness of breathing now causes an unpleasant gasping sensation. The feeling of discomfort is in the chest but is not well localized to any single structure such as the diaphragm or the intercostal muscles.

In contradiction to cardiac dyspnea, shortness of breath at rest is more common in many lung diseases such as asthmatic attacks, bronchitis, pneumonia, pneumothorax, but not in emphysema. Making the distinction between cardiac and pulmonary dyspnea can be extremely difficult. This is not surprising, since the mechanisms may be quite similar in certain circumstances.

A. *Dyspnea Associated with Cardiac Output:* When cardiac output is inadequate to meet the metabolic needs of the body, hyperventilation and dyspnea occur. Pulmonary congestion need not be present, although the dyspnea is similar to that occurring in pulmonary congestion and is quantitatively related to exertion.

B. *Dyspnea due to Pulmonary Edema:* Dyspnea on exertion is the cardinal symptom of pulmonary congestion. It results from a rise in left ventricular end-diastolic pressure or a raised left atrial pressure with a normal left ventricle in mitral valve disease. In both cases, increased pulmonary venous and pulmonary capillary pressures increase the stiffness of the lungs and the work of breathing by decreasing the compliance of the lungs, mainly by causing interstitial pulmonary edema. In addition to the mechanical changes, there is also a reflex autonomic visceral sensation, probably mediated through nonmedullated sensory fibers in the lungs and passing up the vagus nerves to the medulla, which contributes to dyspnea by direct autonomic sensory stimulation. In the early stages of heart disease, dyspnea only occurs with severe exertion, but as pulmonary congestion becomes more severe, permanent changes in the lungs occur. Resting lung compliance is reduced, and increased lymphatic drainage, thickening of interstitial tissues, and other compensatory changes occur. Such changes reduce the chances of acute pulmonary edema and enable the body to tolerate high pulmonary capillary pressures of thickened barriers between the blood in the capillaries and the gas in the alveoli.

C. *Dyspnea in Acute Pulmonary Edema:* When pulmonary congestion is acute and severe, dyspnea occurs with minimal exertion, avid pulmonary edema results as fluid is forced into the alveolar spaces by capillary congestion. This congestion may seriously interfere with gas exchange and cause hypoxia and respiratory acidosis with CO_2 retention.

D. *Dyspnea Associated with other Forms of Heart Disease:* Dyspnea occurs in forms of heart disease other than those involving pulmonary congestion and low cardiac output. In cyanotic congenital heart disease, shunting of venous blood into the systemic circulation lowers arterial oxygen tension and contributes to dyspnea by stimulating the carotid bodies and increasing the ventilation needed for a given work load.

In pulmonary embolism and pulmonary infarction, dyspnea may result from reflex stimulation of medullary centers by impulses from vagal nerve endings in the lungs and pulmonary arteries, Such dyspnea may be in addition to that due to inadequate cardiac output, which has already been described.

Dyspnea Resulting from Chemical Stimuli

Other mechanisms involved in dyspnea include chemical stimuli to ventilation mediated through hypoxia, increase in CO_2 (hypercapnia), and metabolic acidosis. The chemoreceptor cells of the carotid and aortic bodies respond primarily to hypoxia and secondarily to increased CO_2. The central chemosensitive areas in the medulla stimulate respiration primarily in response to acidosis resulting from CO_2 and only secondarily in response to hypoxia. Chemically mediated stimuli to ventilation provide slowly responding and long-lasting control mechanisms and are chiefly involved in controlling depth and rate of breathing rather than causing dyspnea. Hypoxia, as demonstrated by a lowered arterial oxygen tension breathing air at rest or during exercise (PO_2 < 70 mm Hg), is not generally found in dyspneic cardiac patients. Hyperventilation with low pH, and a normal or raised PO_2 is the usual finding. It is caused in cardiac patients by the release of acid metabolites from inadequately perfused tissues rather than by anxiety. Dyspnea also results from acute changes in the permeability of the pulmonary capillaries, as when pulmonary edema develops in heroin overdose, or on exposure to toxic fumes such as chlorine, phosgene, or other noxious gases.

Attacks of Dyspnea

Episodic dyspnea and dyspnea at rest, which is relieved by sitting up (orthopnea), are important indicators of severe disease. The mechanism of' orthopnea involves an increase in pulmonary capillary pressure and a decrease in lung volume when lying flat. Lung compliance decreases and respiratory resistance increases to cause an acute increase in the work of breathing. Paroxysmal dyspnea classically occurs at night, often after a strenuous day or an evening out dancing, or after excessive salt or fluid intake. It characteristically wakes the patient up around 2:00 am and is so clearly relieved by sitting or standing and made worse by lying fiat that a patient who has once experienced this symptom will often never sleep flat in bed again.

In acute pulmonary congestion in bedridden patients, the least exertion, such as eating, use of a bedpan or commode, washing, or the minor excitement of a visitor, may provoke an episode of dyspnea. The dyspnea of acute pulmonary congestion, if not relieved, will progress to acute pulmonary edema, which can cause circulatory collapse, with restlessness, anxiety, apprehension, sweating, tachycardia, tachypnea, and acute respiratory distress.

Dyspnea Associated With High-Altitude

Pulmonary Edema

Dyspnea due to pulmonary edema may occur in persons acutely exposed to hypoxia at altitudes of 2000 m or more. The breathlessness usually comes on in the evening or during the night of the first day at high altitude. The patient often gives a history of unaccustomed exertion during the day. Even previously, acclimatized persons returning to high altitude after a stay at sea level may be affected. Dyspnea, cough, frothy pink sputum, and circulatory collapse may develop if treatment is not forthcoming, and mountain climbers have died from the condition. Oxygen inhalation, aid returning to lower altitude are effective methods of treatment. The causative mechanism is almost certainly increased permeability of the alveolocapillary membrane of the lungs. The left atrial pressure has been shown to be normal person with the condition, and left heart failure is not the primary cause. The chest X-ray shows dramatic changes that disappear rapidly with treatment.

How to Diagnose with Aid of Dyspnea?

Certain features may occasionally help to show that dyspnea is due to specific forms of heart disease. In left ventricular failure, as opposed to pulmonary congestion, dyspnea is often associated with a heavy oppressive substernal discomfort, which tends to merge into angina of effort. Patients with mitral stenosis often complain of angina like pain, but only when there is severe pulmonary hypertension. The distinction between dyspnea alone and angina plus dyspnea on the one hand, and between angina alone and dyspnea plus angina on the other, is difficult for both the patient and the physician to make. Acute left ventricular distention causes both severe discomfort in the chest and dyspnea resulting from acute pulmonary congestion. Similarly, acute imbalance between myocardial oxygen supply and demand often causes an acute rise in left ventricular end-diastolic pressure. In left ventricular failure, dyspnea appears first, and the discomfort never occurs without the dyspnea. The discomfort may radiate like anginal pain and is described as a sensation of heaviness, rather than pain, as in angina. Aortic valve disease, hypertension and cardiomyopathy are the commonest causes of the discomfort. The basic mechanism is an increase in the work required from the left ventricle, and acute left ventricular distention may be involved.

Dyspnea in Normal Subjects

Dyspnea normally limits exercise performance in almost everyone. A person becomes conditioned to a certain level of discomfort arising from some particular task, such as walking up a familiar hill. The ease with which dyspnea is provoked varies with the amount of ventilation required for that task. This in turn depends on a person's physical condition, weight, age, and lifestyle. In sedentary persons, the ability of the circulation to distribute maximum blood flow to the exercising muscles while decreasing perfusion of relatively nonessential vascular beds (e.g. adipose tissue, skin, and viscera) is impaired. A simple exercise program combined with weight reduction will often improve performance adequately within 4–6 weeks.

Dyspnea at Rest

Dyspnea at rest commonly accompanies anxiety. The patient complains that normal breathing is not satisfactory, and it is only by taking deep sighing breaths that relief is obtained. This form of dyspnea is not generally provoked by exertion and is associated with symptoms due to hyperventilation. The deep sighing breaths reduce alveolar and arterial CO_2 resulting in respiratory alkalosis. This provokes cerebral arterial vasoconstriction. Increased anxiety, headaches, dizziness, faintness, and even loss of consciousness can result. In addition, the ionized calcium level decreases with respiratory alkalosis, which can provoke numbness and tingling in fingers and lips, tetany, carpopedal spasm, and convulsions (hyperventilation syndrome). The cycle of anxiety resulting in hyperventilation and causing cerebral symptoms, which in turn increase anxiety, is extremely common and can be broken by the old-fashioned remedy of having the patient rebreathe expired air from a bag (recycling).

Arrhythmias

Supraventricular tachyarrhythmias such as atrial fibrillation rarely cause syncope. The most common cause is bradyarrhythmia, due to sick sinus syndrome or to atrioventricular block, i.e. Stokes-Adams attacks. Drugs, including digoxin, β-blockers and rate-limiting calcium channel blockers, e.g. verapamil, may aggravate attacks. Ventricular tachyarrhythmias often cause syncope or presyncope, especially in patients with impaired left ventricular function.

■ CHEST PAIN

Chest pain is considered to be very important feature of ischemic heart disuse.

Chest pain occurs in many varieties of heart disease and also in noncardiac diseases. Its correct interpretation is occasionally so difficult that it is almost impossible.

Ischemic Cardiac Pain (Angina Pectoris): It is said in a lighter vein that ischemic cardiac pain can occur anywhere from jaw to umbilicus (Fig. 1.2).

The classic ischemic pain of angina pectoris can be either so obvious that no one has the slightest difficulty in recognizing the symptom and arriving at a correct diagnosis, or so atypical that even after complete investigation, significant doubt about the nature of the pain still exists, although the latter is uncommon. The basic mechanism of ischemic pain is an increase in the demand for both coronary blood flow and oxygen delivery, which exceeds the available supply.

A. **Clinical Features:** The original subjective description in the late eighteenth century by William Heberden of his own angina has not been surpassed. Angina of effort is described as a pain or tightness in the chest which is substantial heaviness, burning, and sharp (i.e. severe but not stabbing). It may radiate to the throat, anterior neck and lower jaw (never to the upper jaw), arms, and upper back, but not to the lower spine or below the umbilicus, and rarely to the abdomen

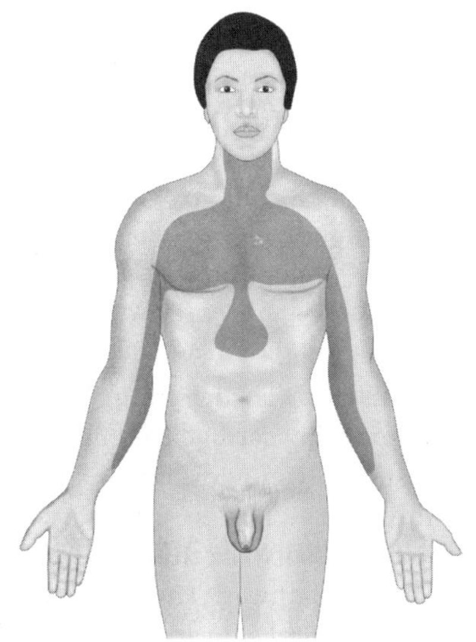

Fig. 1.2: Location of pain in angina pectoris

alone. It more often radiates to the left arm than to the right, and more commonly into both arms than to the right alone. It travels down the ulnar and volar surface of the arm to the wrist but only into the ulnar fingers, never down into the thumb or down the outer surface of the upper arm. Pain may occasionally start in the arms and move to the chest (angina inversus). It occurs more readily after a heavy meal: in cold, windy weather; and with excitement, anger, emotion, or tension. It sometimes comes on more readily with exercise involving the arms. A patient attempting to describe the pain often subconsciously clenches the fists.

B. **Effects of Temperature:** In cold weather, walking against the wind with the face unprotected is likely to provoke anginal pain, cold showers or baths may precipitate pain, and brisk toweling after a shower or bath may also provoke it. The sensory effects of temperature on the face are mediated through the fifth nerve and cause reflex autonomic changes in blood pressure and heart rate. Cold showers raise blood pressure and heart rate. Excitement, mental activity, and physical tension such as simple clenching of the fist raise arterial pressure and heart rate, and increase the work of the heart. When the coronary circulation is severely diseased, even these minor circulatory changes are sufficient to provoke anginal pain. Anginal pain comes on more readily in the presence of fever, anemia, or arrhythmia, both bradycardia and tachycardia.

C. **Mechanism of Cardiac Pain:** The mechanism producing cardiac pain is not clearly understood. Nonmedullated, small sympathetic nerve fibers running with the coronary vessels are thought to provide the afferent pathway. The pain, like other forms of visceral sensation, is referred to the equivalent spinal segments C8 and Tl–5.

Relief of angina following nonspecific surgical procedures such as thoracotomy, mammary artery ligation, and pericardial removal is well recognized but is not consistently found. Although it is thought to be a placebo effect, the severing of afferent autonomic nerves may play a role in relieving pain.

D. **Ischemia without Pain:** Ischemia without pain is often demonstrable on the ECG. In diabetic patients with autonomic nervous system disease, pain may be absent even though ischemia is severe. Chemical substances such as adenosine may provoke pain by stimulating sympathetic nerve endings. Certain compounds such as nicotine provoke visceral sensations that resemble cardiac pain when they are injected into the circulation in normal subjects.

E. **Variant (Prinzmetal's) Angina:** A paradoxical form of angina occurs in some patients as a result of coronary arterial spasm. The pain resembles that of classic angina but occurs at rest rather than on effort. Pain is associated with ST segment elevation rather than depression on the ECG. This form of angina either may be noted in patients with normal coronary arteries when angiography is performed or may occur in the presence of significant coronary atherosclerosis.

Pain of Myocardial Infarction

The pain of myocardial infarction is similar in type and distribution to that of angina of effort, but it is more severe, longer lasting, and associated at times with a feeling of impending death (angor animi) and also with circulatory collapse and shock. The patient may be short of breath, but pain is dominant. Sweating is usually evident.

Pain in Acute Thoracic Disease

Pain similar to that of myocardial infarction also occurs with other acute intrathoracic disorders. Aortic dissection can cause severe chest pain. This frequently starts in the back or radiates to it. Acute pulmonary embolism also causes acute chest pain and shock, which may be indistinguishable from that clue to myocardial infarction. The cause is thought to be sudden acute right ventricular distention that stimulates ventricular receptors whose sensory representation resembles that of the left ventricle. Spontaneous pneumothorax and acute pleurisy, especially at the onset of lobar pneumonia also cause chest pain and must be distinguished from pericardial disease, which causes a pain similar in distribution to other cardiac pains but more related to posture. Like pleural pain, pericardial pain is often worse with respiration, but relief obtained from sitting up and leaning forward or even from crouching on all fours face down is particularly suggestive of pericardial pain. Such maneuvers presumably alter tension on the pericardial sac. Like pleural pain, pericardial pain is often relieved when effusion develops.

Pain Associated with Anxiety States

The most troublesome pain to explain is the non-cardiac pain of anxiety states and effort syndrome. The pain is stabbing, felt at the apex of the heart in the left inframammary region, and associated with a feeling of anxiety, breathlessness, and inability to take a satisfying deep breath (Da Costa's syndrome). It seems to be related to the sympathetic nervous system responses of fright. The more knowledge the patient has of heart disease, the more difficult it may be to interpret such pain, because the description may be unconsciously molded to emphasize or minimize a possible cardiac illness.

Pain Associated with Herpes Zoster

The pain of herpes zoster classically precedes the rash, and this diagnosis should be borne in mind, especially in older persons. The pain is radicular in nature, gripping, tight, and constricting, and it may be severe. The diagnosis, which may

be suspected when hyperesthesia is found in the affected area, becomes obvious when the eruption develops in a few days.

Musculoskeletal Pain

Musculoskeletal pain due to cervical or thoracic spinal bone or joint disease is readily confused with cardiac pain. Dorsal root pain (girdle pain) tends to be gripping and constricting and causes tightness. It is often associated with local tenderness, whereas angina is not. The presence of degenerative changes in spinal radiograms is no positive evidence of a musculoskeletal origin of the pain, any more than ST and T wave changes on the ECG indicate a cardiac origin. Provocation of the pain by movement, jarring, coughing, and sneezing, and relief of pain by means of massage, heat, and manipulation are useful in suggesting a musculoskeletal origin. Tenderness of the anterior rib cage suggests costochondritis (Tietze's syndrome). Pain, which can be easily pointed as localized by finger is usually non-ischemic/non-cardiac.

Abdominal Pain

Abdominal pain sometimes occurs in patients with heart disease, especially in acute, severe right-sided failure. Hepatic distention is usually invoked as the causative mechanism. Abdominal pain also occurs in angina and in myocardial infarction, but the pain is never solely abdominal.

Esophageal spasm and pain associated with hiatal hernia can also be difficult to interpret. The esophagus and the stomach are innervated by the autonomic nervous system and are capable of causing visceral pain having the same area of radiation as the heart. Any disease of the epigastric viscera can cause chest pain, which can be confused with cardiac pain. The pain of gallbladder disease is also difficult to distinguish from cardiac pain, and since gallbladder disease and coronary disease often coexist, accurate diagnosis of the cause of the pain may be extremely difficult.

◼ PALPITATIONS

Abnormal awareness of one's own heartbeats is called palpitations. Awareness of the beating of the heart varies with the sensitivity of the patient and the severity of any disturbance of the force or rhythm of the heartbeat. The variation in these factors is great. Awareness of each ectopic beat or even of normal sinus rhythm may be extremely troublesome to some patients. Others may have an extremely forceful heartbeat owing to free aortic incompetence, or they may be subject to episodes of ventricular or supraventricular tachycardia with heart rates of over 180 beats/min without noticing anything. One must therefore differentiate between awareness of forceful heart action and an arrhythmia when the patient complains of palpitations. Most patients notice irregular rhythms more than they do regular tachycardia, but the more rapid the heartbeat, the more likely the patient is to notice an abnormality. In some cases, arrhythmia is only noticed during exercise when the heart rate is rapid.

Associated Symptoms

An important question is whether the palpitations are accompanied by any other symptoms such as dizziness, chest pain, or dyspnea. The functional effect of an arrhythmia may sometimes be a clue to its cause, as for example in mitral stenosis, in which dyspnea is usually provoked when the arrhythmia occurs.

Examination and Recording of an ECG During an Attack

It is imperative to examine any patient with palpitations and record an ECG during an episode of palpitation. Until this has been done, it is essential to keep an open mind concerning the diagnosis. Palpitations often begin abruptly and cease gradually, and because the sinus

tachycardia resulting from anxiety caused by the arrhythmia subsides only gradually, the patient may not be aware that the arrhythmia itself has stopped. The functional consequences of an episode of palpitations depend on the duration, the rapidity of the heart rate, and the state of the heart before the episode started. A paroxysm of tachycardia at a rate of about 140 beats/min may be well tolerated for a day or two, but any rapid arrhythmia with an acute onset and lasting for more than a week to 10 days is likely to provoke heart failure, even in healthy young persons. In older, sicker patients, especially those with anemia or hypoxia, a shorter time elapses before serious heart failure develops.

◼ DIZZINESS AND SYNCOPE

Dizziness and syncope are difficult symptoms to interpret if the patient's consciousness has been impaired and recollection of the events surrounding the attack is hazy. Dizziness and syncope both occur more commonly as benign manifestations than as symptoms of serious disease. They are most commonly due to noncardiac causes such as epileptic seizures, transient ischemic attacks due to cerebral or carotid vascular disease, and cerebrovascular accidents and vertigo due to vestibular disease rather than cardiac disease. A description of the episode from witnesses is of great value, but much can be learned from the circumstances surrounding the episode, as related by the patient. Dizziness is a frequent but not a necessary precursor of syncope, and one or both occur in three main types of conditions involving the cardiovascular system. The commonest form of cardiac syncope is simple vasovagal fainting resulting from certain autonomic nervous system effects. The next most common is cardiac syncope due to arrhythmia or cardiac standstill, in which the heartbeat does not maintain adequate blood flow to the brain. The least common is syncope on unaccustomed effort, in which the demand for systemic perfusion exceeds the supply during severe stress, and cerebral ischemia ensues. Effort syncope can also occur in severe pulmonary stenosis, in primary pulmonary hypertension, and in severe aortic stenosis.

Fainting Attacks in Tetralogy of Fallot

A specific form of syncope occurs in patients with tetralogy of Fallot in whom infundibular obstruction is present. Spasm of the muscle of the outflow tract of the right ventricle results in an acute decrease in pulmonary blood flow. Right-to-left shunting of blood through the ventricular septal defect into the aorta increases as a result, and acute severe arterial hypoxemia occurs, leading to loss of consciousness. The factors precipitating the infundibular spasm are not known. Beta-blocking agents such as propranolol are the most effective remedies. The condition is most commonly seen in children but can occur in adults.

Carotid Sinus Syncope

Another rare cause of syncope is excessive sensitivity of the carotid sinus baroreceptor mechanism. Extreme bradycardia and peripheral vasodilatation may occur in response to minor mechanical stimulation of the neck, as in sharp turning of the head or pressure on the neck from too tight a collar. The condition is generally seen in older atherosclerotic men.

Cough Syncope

Syncope sometimes follows a bout of coughing. In this case, the repeated large (> 100 mm Hg) increases in intrathoracic pressure reduce systemic venous return enough to lower the systemic arterial pressure to levels of 50 mm Hg or less. Syncope results from inadequate cerebral perfusion. Either continuous or intermittent coughing spasms may cause these effects, which are commonest in middle-aged male smokers.

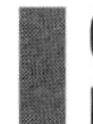 **OTHER SYMPTOMS OF HEART DISEASE**

Cough and Hemoptysis

Hemoptysis may occasionally be the first symptom of heart disease, and since there can be no hemoptysis without cough, cough is technically the presenting svrnptom. Mitral valve stenosis is the commonest condition in which hemoptysis is the presenting manifestation, and pulmonary congestion, frank pulmonary hemorrhage due to a ruptured vessel, and pulmonary infarction account for almost all cases. Cough without hemoptysis also occurs in any condition causing pulmonary congestion, and cough on exercise is sometimes seen in patients with mitral stenosis. Dry and unproductive cough is usually the earliest manifestation of impending pulmonary edema and precedes the profuse, watery, frothy pink sputum seen in the fully developed picture of acute pulmonary edema.

Cough may also occur as a manifestation of pressure on the bronchial tree in patients with cardiovascular disease. Left atrial enlargement may compress the left main bronchus in patients with mitral valve disease, and it may irritate the recurrent laryngeal nerve on the left side as it hooks under the aorta. Enlarging aortic aneurysms involving the aortic arch and tumors involving the heart may also cause cough when they compress mediastinal structures. Cough that occurs when the patient lies flat and is relieved when the patient sits up is particularly suggestive of pressure on the bronchial tree.

Fatigue

Fatigue is the most difficult cardiac symptom to evaluate. Whereas other symptoms of heart disease have associated outward manifestations. Fatigue is entirely subjective. Although it is sometimes due to heart disease, fatigue is far more frequently due to noncardiac causes. Fatigue as a cardiac symptom is almost never of diagnostic value except as an indication of low cardiac output. It is rarely the first or the only symptom of significant organic heart disease, although it is a prominent symptom of neurocirculatory asthenia (Da Costa's syndrome). It commonly accompanies severe long-standing heart disease, especially chronic valvular disease with persistent right heart failure and low cardiac output. It is seen in patients with severe coronary artery disease after myocardial infarction, in mitral stenosis with marked increase in pulmonary vascular resistance, and in primary pulmonary hypertension. Dehydration due to excessive diuretic therapy and potassium depletion are two additional contributing factors.

Nocturia and Polyuria

Nocturia is occasionally the earliest symptom of raised left atrial pressure in left ventricular failure or mitral stenosis. The exact mechanism is not known, but transfer of fluid from the legs to the thorax when the patient lies down may play a part. Reflex connections have been demonstrated between left atrial receptors and the central nervous system, and the efferent pathway is known to involve the kidneys. Nocturia implies the passage of an abnormally large amount of urine at night, rather than an increased frequency of micturition at night, as occurs in prostatic disease. In the healthy state, the cardiac output is sufficient to provide adequate renal blood flow during the day, and urine flow at night is therefore conveniently reduced to a minimum. It may be that in early heart failure this mechanism breaks down because of inadequate cardiac output. There is also a connection between cardiac function and urinary output in patients with paroxysmal tachycardia due to any cause. Some patients note an increased urinary volume within 15–30 minutes of the start of tachycardia. The urine is of low specific gravity. The possibility of a

reflex mechanism involving left atrial distention remains to be proved.

Squatting

Exertional dyspnea that is relieved by squatting during recovery from exercise strongly suggests the diagnosis of tetralogy of Fallot. Squatting is seldom seen after puberty. It is a convenient means of increasing systemic venous return by lowering the patient's center of gravity and counteracting any tendency for blood to pool in the veins of the legs and pelvis. The central blood volume and pulmonary blood flow, both are increased by squatting. It has been shown that it is the change in the amount of venous return and not the change in posture which is important, because squatting in water has no hemodynamic effect. Thus, in tetralogy of Fallot, squatting increases the arterial pressure and provides more blood flow to the lungs by decreasing the right-to-left shunt across the ventricular defect. It provides more pulmonary blood flow and a greater left ventricular inflow and also raises the arterial oxygen saturation by reducing the shunting effect. A similar result can be obtained by lying down, but children find it easier to squat after exertion. It is the pooling of blood in the legs in the upright position after stopping exercise that is the primary problem; if this does not occur, as in patients with a large pulmonary blood volume, the benefit from squatting is not seen.

Surprisingly squatting does not help when patient is in water.

Hoarseness

Hoarseness as a manifestation of heart disease is seldom, if ever, a presenting symptom. It occurs in cardiac patients with gross left atrial enlargement in mitral valve disease, in giant left atrium, and in aortic dissection. All of these conditions cause pressure on the left recurrent laryngeal nerve and result in hoarseness. Hoarseness is also seen in patients with myxedema, in whom it may be the first clue to diagnosis.

Edema

Since edema due to cardiac disease is a result of right heart failure, it is seldom seen early, because right heart failure is a late development in heart disease. A complaint of edema as a primary symptom implies a noncardiac cause such as venous stasis, thrombophlebitis. nephrotic syndrome, lymphedema, or idiopathic edema. Edema is seldom seen in patients with congestive heart failure under good medical control now that effective diuretic therapy is available. Right heart failure can be surprisingly severe, with hepatic enlargement, ascites, and a raised venous pressure, but no significant pitting edema of the ankles.

Cyanosis

Cyanosis is more a sign than a symptom, although patients do occasionally complain of blueness of the extremities, face, and lips. Cyanosis may be peripheral and associated with a low cardiac output, peripheral vasoconstriction, and a feeling of coldness. In this case, the blueness is due to a high concentration of reduced hemoglobin in the blood in the veins of the skin, and arterial saturation is normal. In true central cyanosis, the arterial oxygen saturation is reduced because of right-to-left shunting or lung disease. In this case, the patient's extremities are often warm, or, if they are made warm, the blue color does not disappear.

Loss of Weight (Cardiac Cachexia)

Loss of weight is not a presenting symptom of heart disease, but it does occur in chronically ill cardiac patients, especially when the cardiac output is low. It is probably related to secondary anorexia. The patient characteristically loses weight from the limbs and accentuates fluid in the abdomen. It is difficult to establish the true extent of the cachexia, because the accumulation of fluid tends to maintain total body weight.

FUNCTIONAL AND THERAPEUTIC CLASSIFICATION OF HEART DISEASE

The patient's overall disability is conventionally expressed in terms of the New York Heart Association's criteria for functional capacity and therapeutic class.

Functional Capacity (Four Classes)

Class I: No limitation of physical activity.' Ordinary physical activity does not cause undue fatigue, palpitation, dyspnea, or anginal pain.

Class II: Slight limitation of physical activity. Comfortable at rest but ordinary physical activity results in fatigue, palpitation, dyspnea, or anginal pain.

Class III: Marked limitation of physical activity. Comfortable at rest, but less than ordinary activity causes fatigue, palpitation, dyspnea, or anginal pain.

Class IV: Unable to carry on any physical activity without discomfort. Symptoms of cardiac insufficiency, or of the anginal syndrome, may be present even at rest. If any physical activity is undertaken, discomfort is increased.

While this classification gives a good overall indication of the patient's status, many physicians prefer to subdivide class II into classes IIa and IIb. In class IIa, the patient can keep up with others walking on the flat but has limitation on more severe exercise such as climbing stairs. In class IIb, the patient has slight limitation on all forms of physical activity.

Therapeutic Classification (Five Classes)

Class A: Physical activity need not be restricted.

Class B: Ordinary physical activity need not be restricted, but unusually severe or competitive efforts should be avoided.

Class C: Ordinary physical activity should be moderately restricted, and more strenuous efforts should be discontinued.

Class D: Ordinary physical activity should be markedly restricted.

Class E: Patient should be at complete rest, confined to bed or chair.

■ BIBLIOGRAPHY

1. Barcroft H, McMichael J. Posthaemorrhagic fainting study by cardiac output and forearm flow. Lancet. 1944;1:489-91.
2. Grover RF, Hultgren HN, Hartley LH. Pathogenesis of acute pulmonary edema at high altitude. In: Central Hemodynamics and Gas Exchange. Giuntini C (editor). Minerva Medica, 1971.p.409.
3. Heberden W. Commentaries on the History and Cure of Diseases. London, 1802.
4. Herrick JB. Clinical features of sudden obstruction of the coronary arteries. JAMA. 1912;59:2015-20.
5. Hultgren HN, Lopez CE, Lundberg E, Miller H. Physiologic studies of pulmonary edema at high altitude. Circulation. 1964;29:393-408..
6. Johnson AD, Detweiler JH. Coronary spasm, variant angina, and recurrent myocardial infarctions. Circulation. 1977;55(6):947-50.
7. Mcilroy MB. Breathlessness in cardiovascular disease. In: Manchester Symposium on Breathlessness. Blackwell, 1966. pp. 187-202.
8. O'Donnell TV, Mcilroy MB. The circulatory effects of squatting. Am Heart J. 1962;64:347-56.
9. Parry CH. An Inquiry into the Symptoms and Causes of the Syncope Anginosa, commonly Called Angina Pectoris: Illustrated by Dissections. London, 1799.
10. Sharpey-Schafer EP. The mechanism of syncope after coughing. Br Med J 1953;2:860-3.

Chapter 2

Physical Examination

Despite rapid advances in diagnostic equipment and technology, physical examination still is considered to be a very important and handy skill for diagnostic purposes. One should not feel helpless if sophisticated diagnostic machines are not available at times especially in rural area.

It is important to emphasize that examination of the cardiac patient is not confined to those parts of the body in which manifestations of cardiac disease are most commonly seen. Physicians should remember that cardiac disease can be associated with many diseases and that clues to the existence of non-cardiac disorders which simulate, complicate, or merely coexist with heart disease may be apparent on methodic physical examination.

APPROACH TO THE PHYSICAL EXAMINATION

The general appearance and behavior of the patient are noted as the medical history is recorded. Similarly, the history-taking process may continue during the physical examination. The patient may be questioned about any findings and asked about awareness of signs and duration of such manifestations.

Examination of the patient usually starts from the head and proceeds downward. Inspection precedes palpation, percussion, and auscultation. The cardiologist traditionally feels the patient's pulse while carrying out the preliminary inspection, and many physicians start by recording the vital signs—pulse, temperature, and respiration—and blood pressure.

Patient can be asked how long he had been noting clubbing/agenesis/nodules.

The Radial Pulse

Palpation of the pulse wave that results from transmission of the pressure wave down the artery is classically performed on the patient's right wrist, with the examiner using the first three fingers of the right hand (Figs 2.1 and 2.4). The frequency, regularity, amplitude, rate upstroke, and volume of the radial pulse require only one finger for their evaluation. Pulse volume (small or large) depends mainly on the pulse pressure and gives a rough indication of stroke volume. Thus, the "small" pulse of server mitral stenosis contrasts with the "large", jerky pulse seen in patients with mitral incompetence. In aortic stenosis, the rate of travel of the wave is slow: the "pulsus tardus", this condition means that the pulse takes longer to pass under the examiner's fingers. The ease with which the pulse can be obliterated is felt by compressing the artery with the proximal finger and palpating with the other two in order to ascertain when the wave has disappeared. It is a rough indication of the systolic arterial pressure and is less accurate than the measurement obtained by sphygmomanometry. The thickness of the undistended arterial wall can be felt using the middle finger to palpate while the proximal and distal fingers simultaneously occlude the vessel. It gives an indication of the degree of atherosclerosis.

Other Pulses

It is important to feel the pulse bilaterally to check for differences in timing and intensity (Figs 2.2A and B). Brachial, radial, carotid, femoral, popliteal, and posterior tibial pulses are usually examined routinely. By this means, the physician may obtain clues about peripheral vascular disease, aortic dissection, and coarctation of the aorta. The closer the vessel lies to the heart, the more reliable the pulse is as an indicator of aortic pressure wave characteristics. Thus, the carotid arterial pulse is best for assessment of aortic valve disease. If there is a prominent pulse in the neck or if coarctation of the aorta is suspected for any other reason, it is important to feel the radial and femoral pulses simultaneously (Fig. 2.1D). In normal subjects, the 2 pulses are clinically synchronous, whereas in coarctation of the aorta the femoral pulse is felt up to 0.15 sec after the radial.

Measurement Technique in the Arms (Figs 2.3, 2.5 and 2.6)

Indirect measurement of the systemic arterial pressure is conventionally performed using a sphygmomanometer on the right arm. A 12.5 cm cuff is wrapped around the upper arm and connected to a mercury or aneroid manometer. The arm is placed at heart level and the cuff is inflated to a level above the systolic pressure. The absence of a radial pulse is checked at the wrist. The cuff is slowly deflated (around 2 mm/beat) while the examiner feels the radial pulse. The pressure level at which the pulse is first felt is noted, and the cuff is reinflated. The cuff is then deflated a second time, with the examiner listening over the brachial artery with the stethoscope. The pressure level at which a sound is first heard over the artery is recorded as the systolic pressure. As deflation of the cuff continues, the sound arising from the vessel wall increases in intensity, decreases, becomes muffled, and finally disappears, differences of opinion exist about the accuracy of considering the muffing or disappearance of sound as an indication of the diastolic pressure. Because the appropriate world cardiologic governing bodies are still undecided about whether it is the muffing of the sounds or their disappearance that is the "correct" level to use, both should be recorded. Correlation between direct arterial pressure measurement and sphygmonanometry has shown reasonable agreement between the two methods, especially in normal subjects, but the differences are sometimes marked in individual cases.

Blood pressure should be measured in both the standing and the supine positions in patients who might have hypotension or hypertension, and the pulse rate should always be measured and recorded along with the pressure. Blood pressure should be measured in both arms when the patient is first seen. On subsequent visits, it is taken in the right arm, except when the pulse in that arm is significantly reduced, as, for example, after a Blalock-Tausing operation for tetralogy of Fallot. The site of the measurement and position of the patient should be recorded.

Artifacts in Measurement

Artifacts in indirect measurement occur when the arm is large in relation to the cuff; when a patient has aortic incompetence, in which the indirectly measured diastolic pressure is usually falsely low: and when the patient is in shock. An erroneously low systolic pressure may be obtained in some hypertensive patients in whom the systolic pressure in not checked by palpation. An "auscultatory gap" may be present in such patients and in those with aortic stenosis and localized arteriosclerosis. The auscultatory gap is a range of pressures over which arterial sounds are absent even though arterial flow is present and the cuff pressure is not above the arterial pressure.

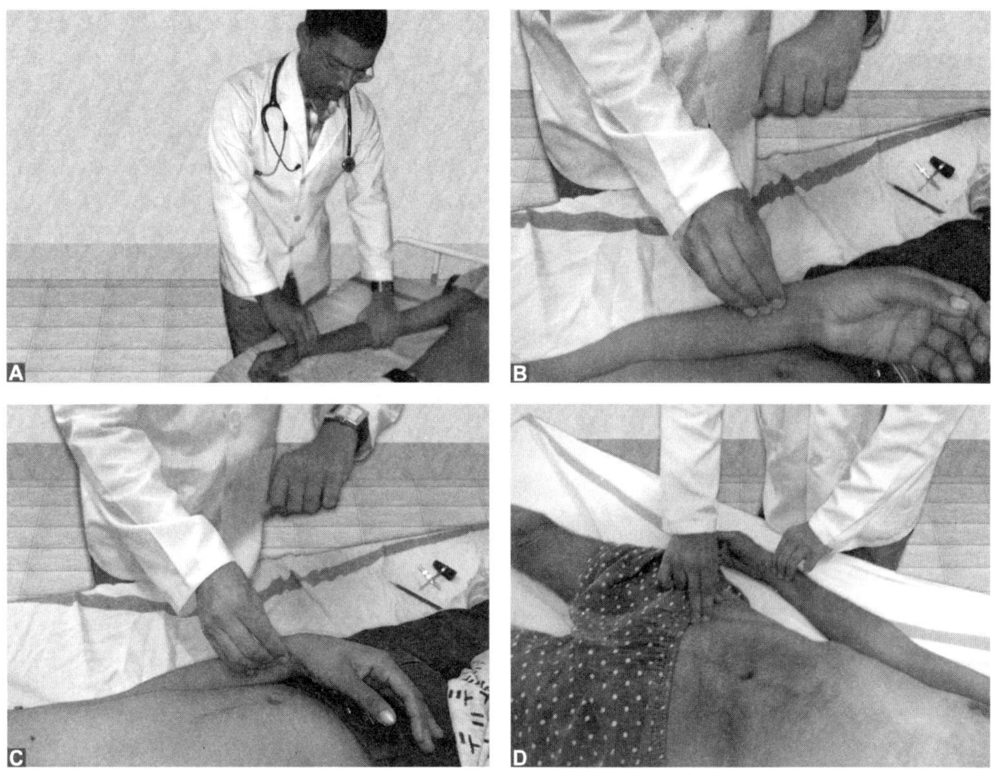

Figs 2.1A to D: Radial pulse, radiofemoral delay

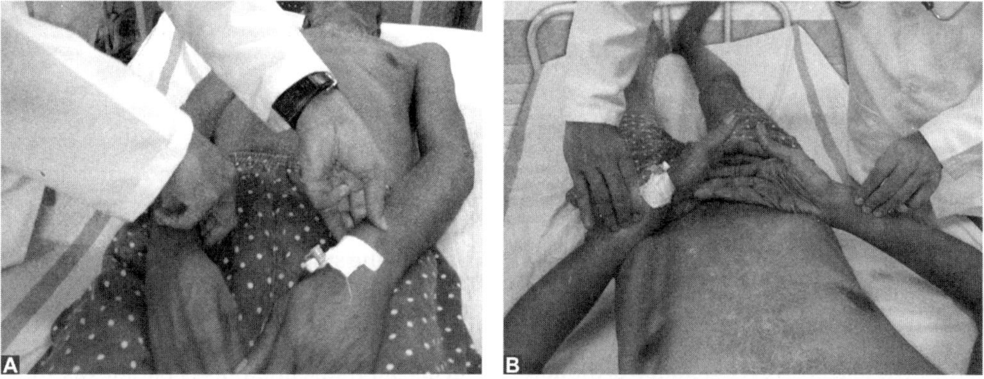

Figs 2.2A to B: Comparison of both, radial arteries

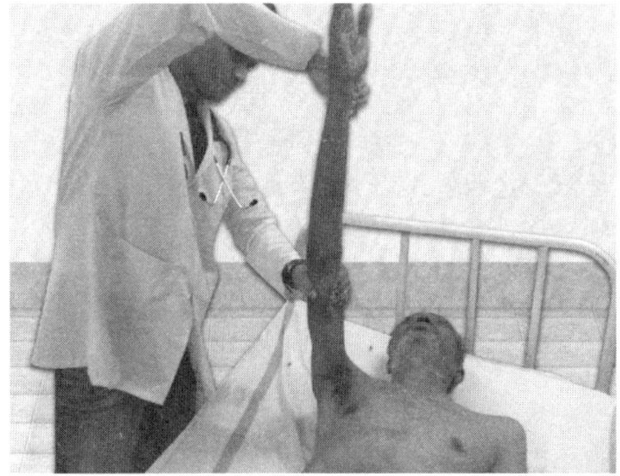

Fig. 2.3: Water hammer pulse

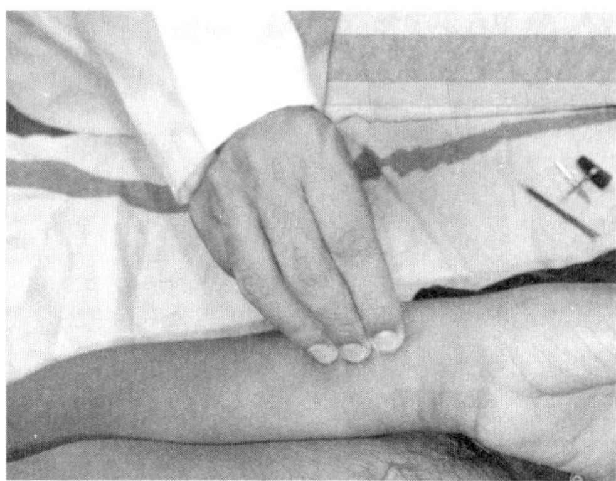

Fig. 2.4: Three finger technique for pulse

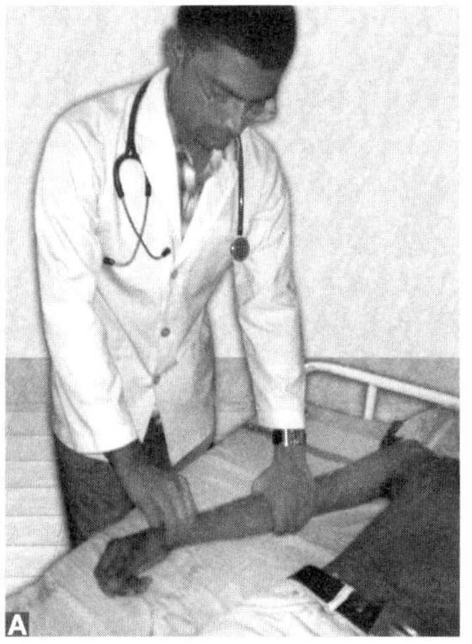

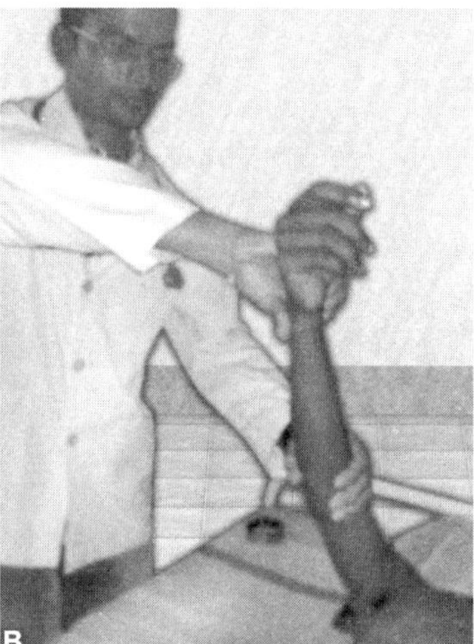

Figs 2.5A and B: Technique for water hammer pulse

Blood Pressure in the Legs

The measurement of arterial pressure in both arms and both legs is advocated by some as a routine measure. If the leg pressure is to be measured, a special wide (20 cm) cuff in sued: such a cuff is also needed for patients with thick or fat arms. The diagnosis of coarctation of the aorta is usually made on other grounds. In difficult cases, simultaneous brachial and femoral arterial tracings during exercise may be needed.

Pulses Alternans and Pulsus Paradoxus

Pulsus alternans and pulsus paradoxus should be sought when the blood pressure is measured.

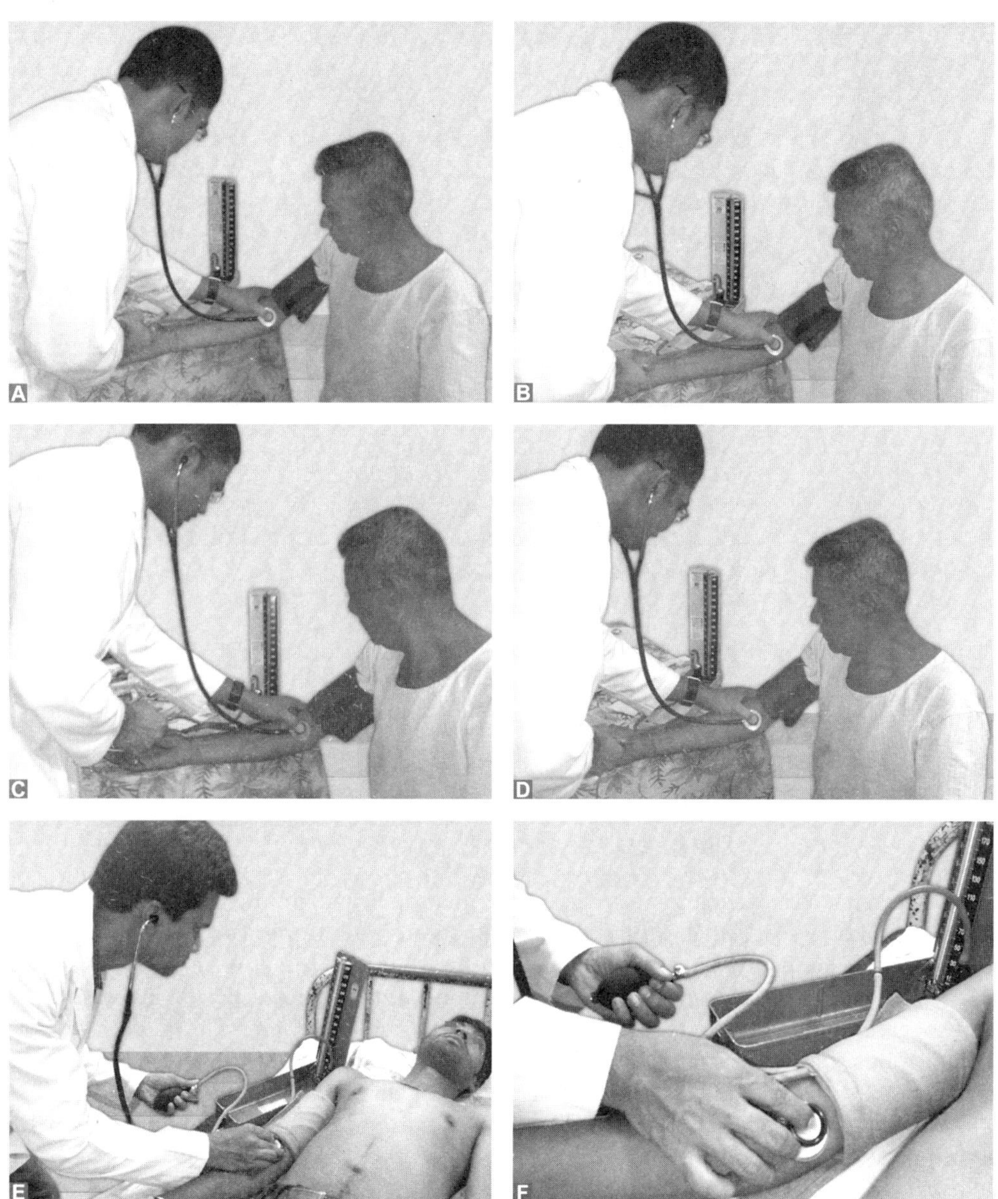

Figs 2.6A to F: Measurement of blood pressure

In pulsus alternans, every other heartbeat produces a higher systolic pressure. The mechanism is unknown although many theories have been proposed, and the finding, which is seen in left ventricular failure, carries a poor prognosis, especially if the heart rate is slow.

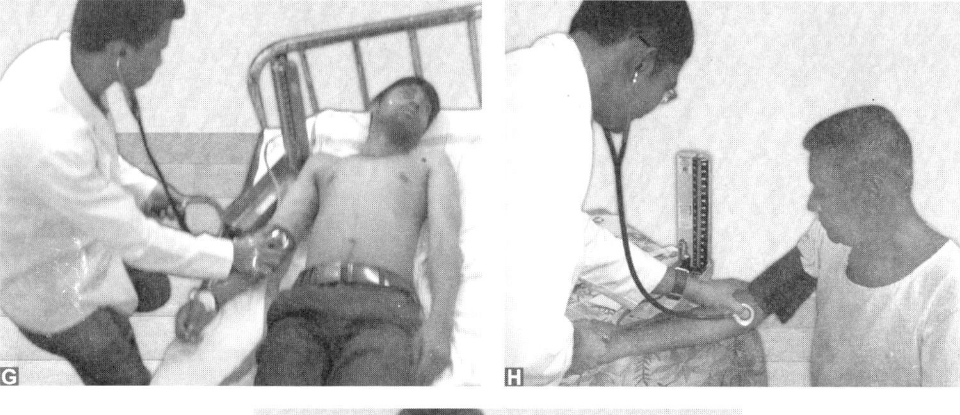

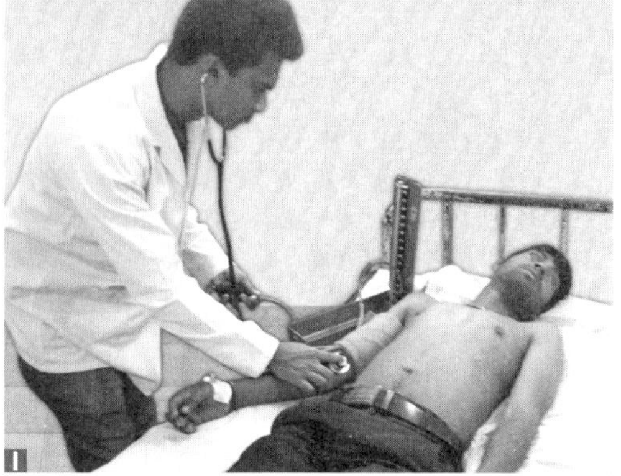

Figs 2.6G to I: Measurement of blood pressure

Pulsus paradoxus is principally associated with pericardial disease in which cardiac filling is compromised. The abnormality shown in right and left ventricular pressure tracings consists of an exaggeration of the normal respiratory fluctuation in systolic pressure. The arterial pressure (systolic, diastolic, and mean) normally falls by a few mm Hg when intrathoracic negative pressure increases during inspiration. If the systolic fall amounts to greater than 10 mm Hg (or more than 10% of the systolic pressure). Pulsus paradoxus is present. The phenomenon can be due to an increase in the amplitude of intrathoracic pressure fluctuations resulting from changes in the mechanical properties of the lungs, as occurs in large pneumothorax, pleural effusion, or obstructive lung disease. It is more commonly due to pericardial disease, especially cardiac tamponade, as fluid accumulated in the pericardial cavity in the course of pericardial effusion, the intrapericardial pressure rises. If the fluid is formed more rapidly than the pericardium can stretch, the rise in pressure may be sufficient to compress the heart in diastole. If pericardium has time to stretch, and cardiac tamponade does not occur.

Cardiac tamponade occurs when the pericardial pressure reaches the level of the diastolic pressure in the heart. Since the right-sided pressure is lower than those of the left, the right is the first to be compressed. In tamponade, the maintenance of cardiac volume depends on the level of the venous pressure (right- and left-sided), and the 2 ventricles compete for blood with which to fill in diastole. Respiration has a marked effect on homodynamics, with inspiration favoring the right ventricle both by increasing its filing, volume, and output and also by pooling blood in the lungs, decreasing left-sided venous return and occasionally displacing the ventricular septum in severe cases. Conversely, on expiration, the extra blood passes from the lungs to the left ventricle as the right ventricle is compressed and left-sided output enhanced. Pulsus paradoxus is the most obvious clinical sign of this process. It does not occur in cardiac tamponade until the pericardial pressure has risen to the level of the right atrial pressure, and it disappears when sufficient fluid is withdrawn to make the pericardial pressure lower than the atrial pressure. The pericardial pressure must rise to equal or exceed that in both the left and the right ventricles before pulsus paradoxus occurs. If the left ventricle is hypertrophied, as in hypertension associated with chronic renal disease, it is less readily compressed by pericardial effusion, and right ventricular tamponade can occur before left ventricular tamponade. Pulses parardoxus does not occur until filing of both ventricles is impaired. The reciprocal effects of respiration are an essential part of the mechanism in pericardial tamponade.

In pericardial constriction there is little or no pericardial space, and pulsus paradoxus is not always seen (it is present in about half of cases), However, it can occur when the heart is encased in an unyielding shell of tissue, when there is insufficient space within the pericardium to accommodate the inspiratory increase in venous return, an increase in right heart volume can only occur at the expense of left heart volume. Blood thus pools in the lungs during inspiration and pulsus paradoxus results.

▌ EXAMINATION OF ORGANS AND REGIONS OTHER THAN THE HEART

Examination of organs of the body than the heart can provide important clues in the diagnosis of heart disease, clinical findings and the symptoms and signs that may be noted on examination of various body structures are noted below.

Eyes (Figs 2.7A and B, Fig. 2.8, Figs 2.16 to 2.20, 2.24 and 2.27)

Examination of the eyes may disclose petechial hemorrhages, which are evidence of embolism, or conjunctival pallor due to anemia. Examination of the ocular fundus is particularly important in patients with atherosclerotic vascular disease and especially in cases of hypertension. Direct visual examination of small arteries and arterioles in the fundus offers an important opportunity to assess the condition of the blood vessels, the retina, and the optic disk. Hemorrhages and embolic phenomena (Roth spots) can also be seen in the retinas of patients with infective endocarditis.

Mouth (Figs 2.7C and D)

The mucous membranes of the mouth and tongue can demonstrate reduced arterial oxygen saturation by their bluish color, but this physical sign is difficult to interpret and should always be checked by measuring arterial oxygen levels.

Ears (Fig. 2.25)

Inspection of the earlobe may reveal a deep crease in the lobe of the ear at the site. Ear creases are associated with age and are present in most people over age 60. However, their occurrence in younger people is associated with a high incidence of premature atherosclerotic changes involving the cerebral, coronary, or aortoiliac vessels.

Neck

The venous pulse and pressure, the nature of the carotid pulse, and the presence of a goiter are sought in the examination of the neck. Accentuated pulsations of the carotid arteries are seen in coarctation of the aorta and aortic incompetence. In aortic stenosis, the carotid pulse is slow rising and of small amplitude. Marked pulsation in the base of the neck on the right side is seen in elderly atherosclerotic

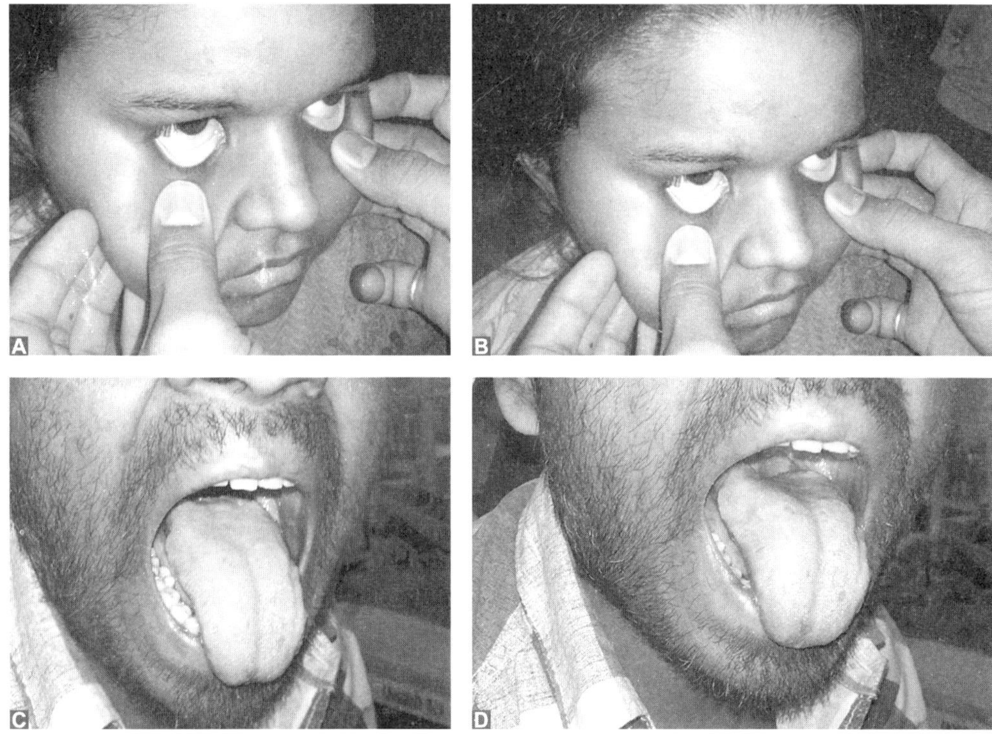

Figs 2.7A to D: Pallor in eyes and tongue

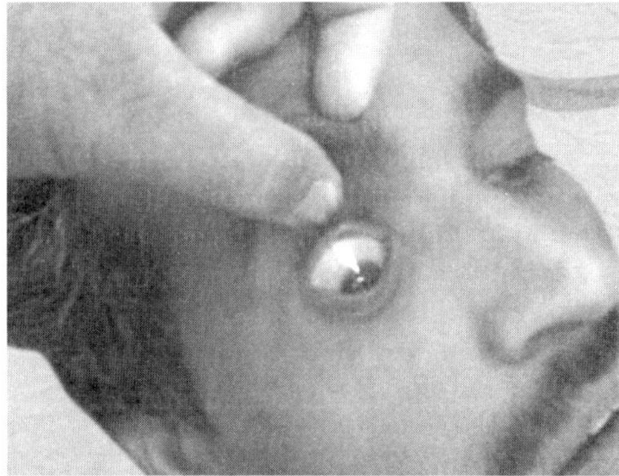

Fig. 2.8: Icterus

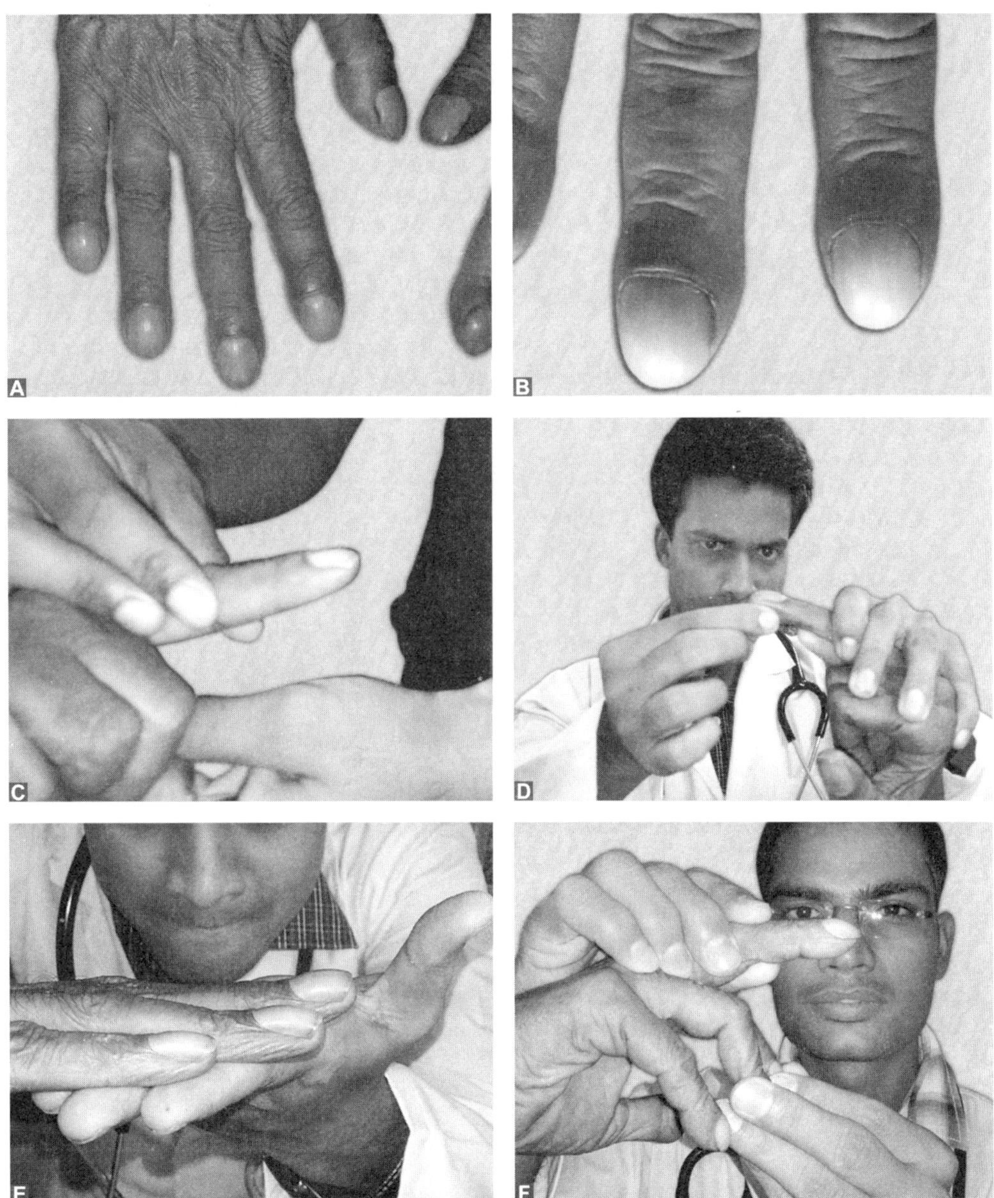

Figs 2.9A to F: Examination for clubbing

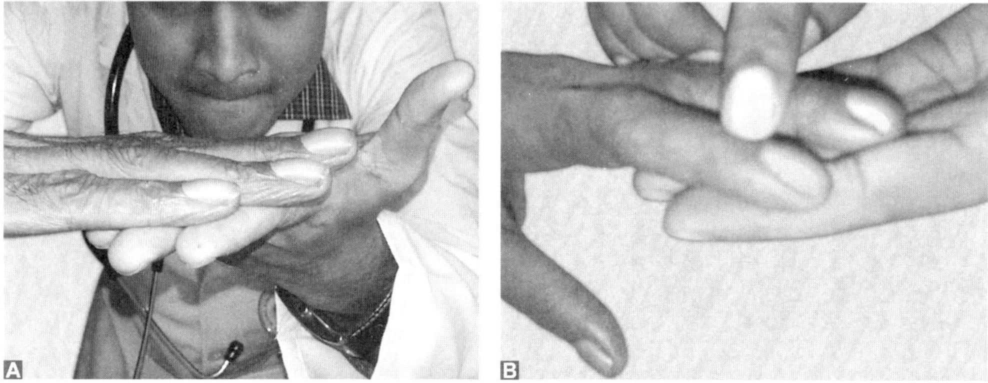

Figs 2.10A to B: Clubbing of fingers

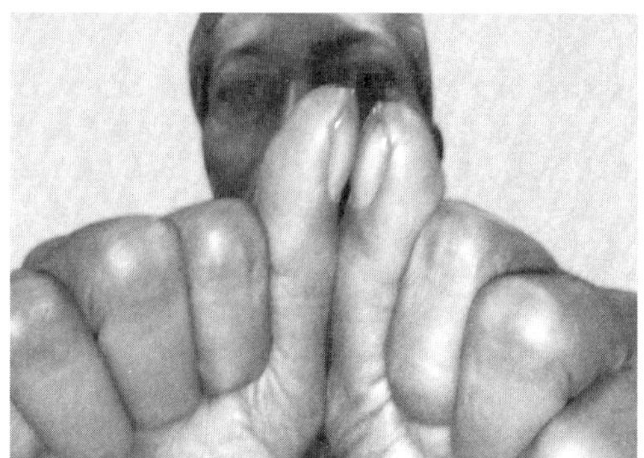

Fig. 2.11: Demonstration for clubbing of fingers

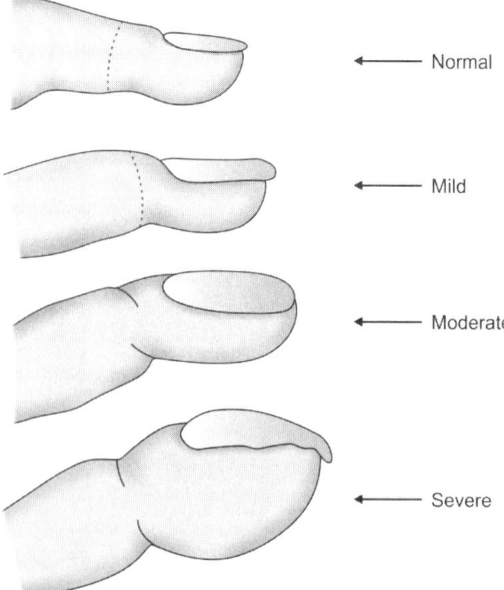

Fig. 2.12: Various grades of clubbing

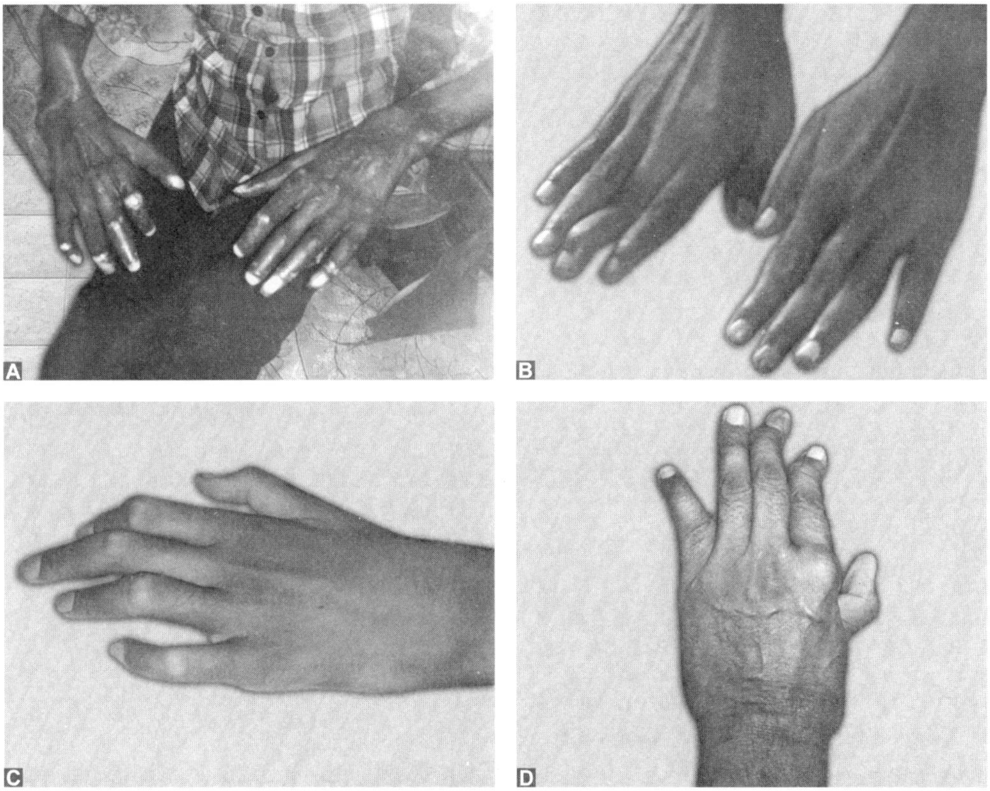

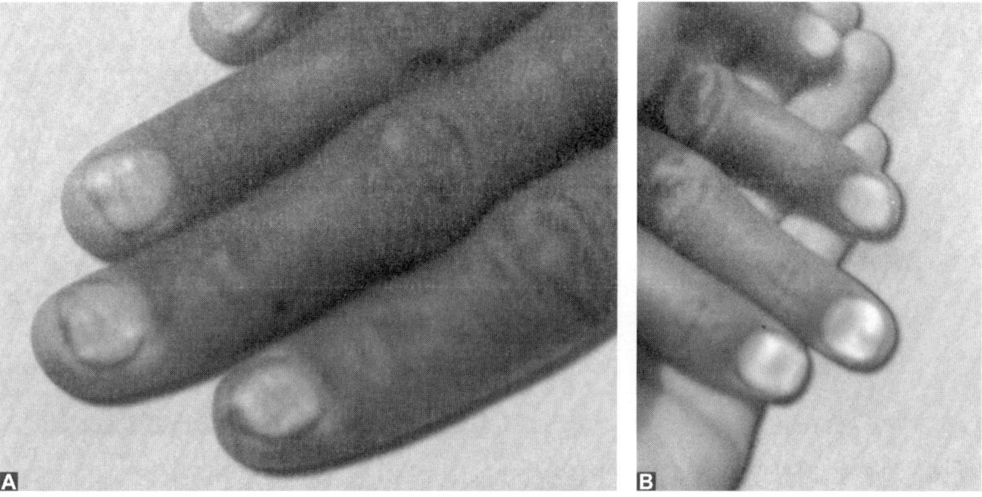

Figs 2.13A to D: Rheumatoid arthritis

Figs 2.14A and B: Koilonychia

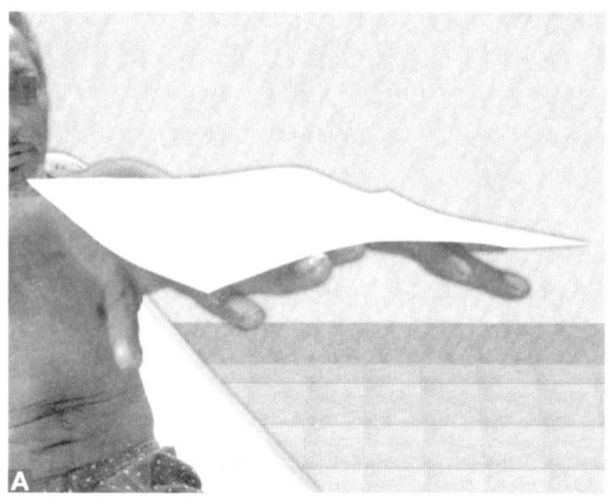
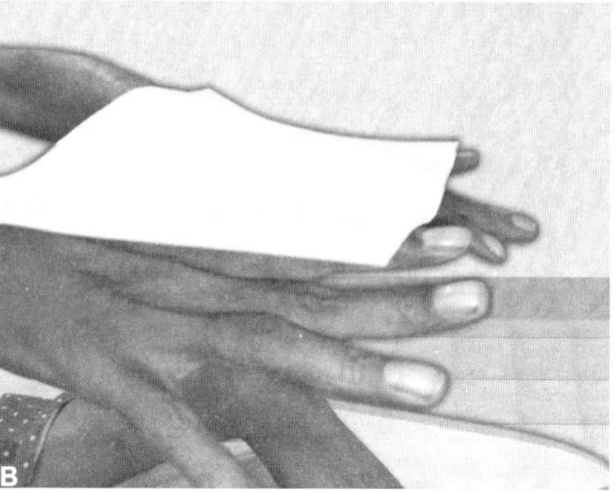
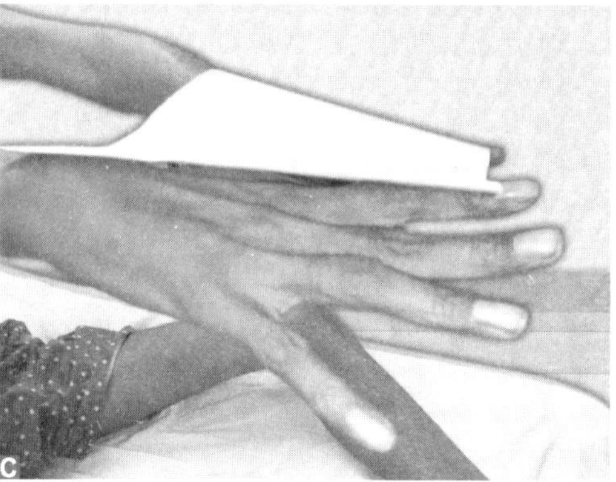

Figs 2.15A to C: Demonstration of tremors

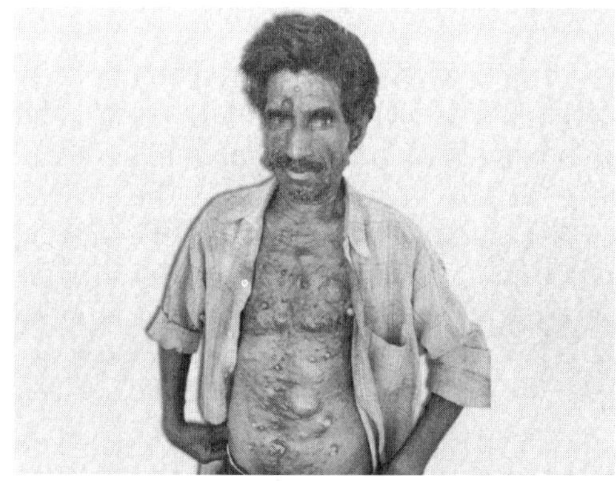

Fig. 2.16: Neurofibromatosis (Hypertension)

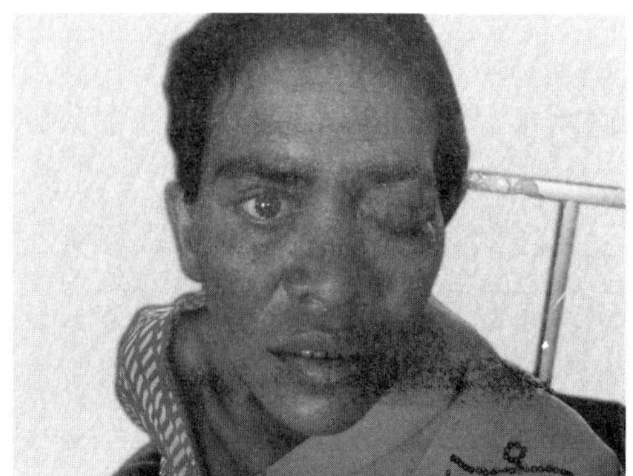

Fig. 2.17: Horner's Syndrome

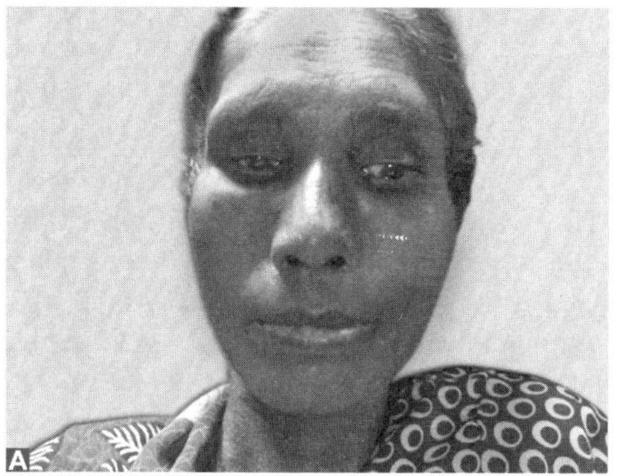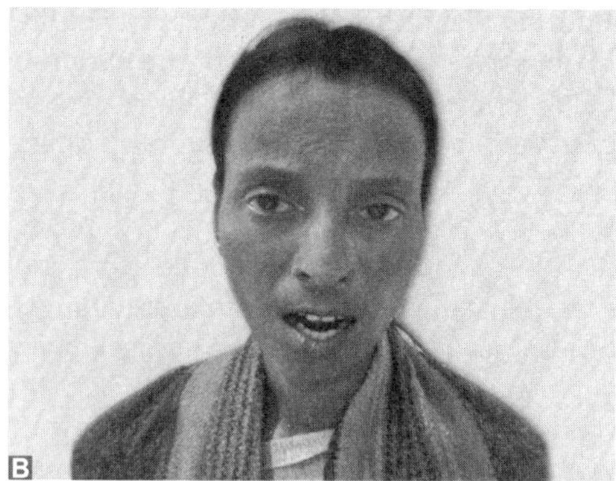

Figs 2.18A and B: Scleroderma

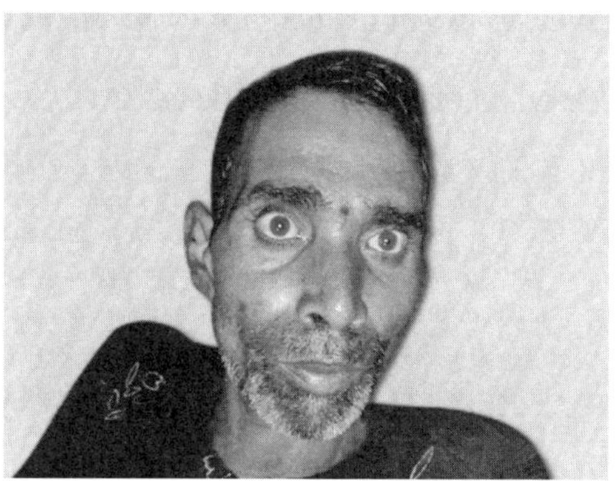

Fig. 2.19: Hyperthyroidism

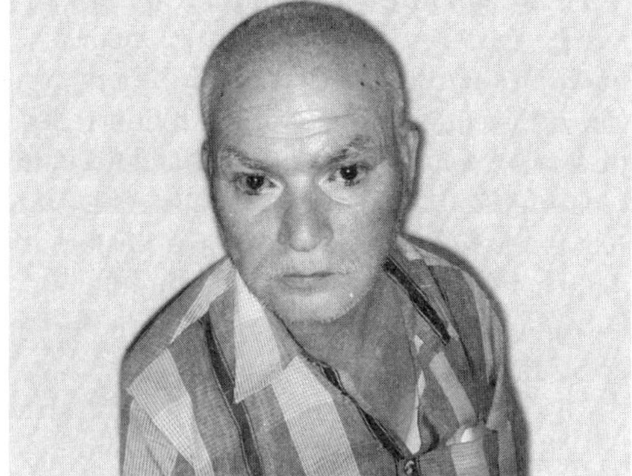

Fig. 2.20: Cholesterol deposits near eyelids

people. It is due to kinking of the right carotid artery resulting from dilatation of the aortic arch, which makes the aorta take a higher course in the mediastinum. This benign condition is more common in women.

Venous Pulse and Venous Pressure (Figs 2.21 to 2.23)

The level of the venous pressure and the nature of the venous pulse are perhaps the most important observations to be made in the examination of the neck. The internal jugular vein should be examined because it lies deep to the sternocleidomastoid muscle and is in free communication with the right atrium. The external jugular vein is often easier to see, but it may be constricted as it passes through the fascial planes of the neck and may give an inaccurate assessment of venous events. The positioning of the patient is most important in examining the veins in the neck. The angle at which the patient is supported in the bed should be adjusted to bring the meniscus of blood in the vein to a level between the clavicles and the angle of the jaw. The higher the venous pressure, the more erect the patient should be, patients with severe venous congestion may have to stand up and breathe in deeply in order to bring the level of the meniscus into view. The head should be comfortably supported in order to relax the neck muscles. Any movement of the earlobes should be noted, because this is always due to venous rather than arterial pulsation. Timing of the venous waves against the carotid pulse is carried out by feeling the artery on the opposite side of the neck or by listening to the heart, and not by feeling the radial pulse. Interpretation of the pulse wave pattern is sometimes facilitated by observing when the venous pressure falls. The first venous trough, the X descent, coincides with the carotid arterial pulse. Distinguishing arterial from venous pulses in the neck can be difficult. Venous pulses are usually not palpable; they are diffusely expansile and influenced by respiration.

Some authorities advocate exerting pressure over the abdomen to distend the neck veins. They maintain that the magnitude of the resulting venous distention (hepatojugular reflux) reflects the level of venous congestion. We believe that hepatojugular reflux is especially marked in right heart failure, and that proper positioning of the patient, relaxation with the mouth open, and quiet normal breathing are more important factors in evaluating venous pressure.

Direct bedside assessment of right atrial pressure requires skill and practice, but it can obviate the need for central venous pressure measurement, which requires use of catheter. The level of the venous pressure is most important in distinguishing cardiac failure with edema and ascites form hepatic or renal disease with similar findings. Unfortunately, it is often in those patients with highest venous pressures that the examiner fails to note the raised pressure due to its invisibility.

Normal Venous Pulse

The positive waves are a, c, and v, and the troughs are X1, X2, and Y. The a wave is due to atrial contraction. It follows the P wave of the ECG and is absent in atrial fibrillation. The origin of the c wave is more controversial. It was originally noted in tracing of the venous pressure in the neck and attributed to the effects of carotid arterial pulsation. When it was also observed in right atrial pressure tracings, however, this explanation became untenable. It is now thought to be due to bulging of the tricuspid valve back into the atrium at the start of ventricular systole. The v wave is associated with atrial filling; pressure in the atrium rises to the v peak and falls as the tricuspid valve pens and the atrium empties into the ventricle. The X1 and X2 troughs are attributed to descent of the base of the heart during ventricular systole. The backward bulging of the valve interrupts this process to produce the c wave. The c wave is not always seen. The y descent to the y trough is due to atrial emptying, and its rate is influenced by stenosis or insufficiency of the atrioventricular valve.

Abnormal or Exaggerated Waves

1. *Cannon waves:* The magnitude of the a wave resulting from atrial contraction varies with the P-R interval. The a waves associated with these beats are larger and are referred to as cannon waves because of their explosive appearance when seen in the neck. The largest cannon waves are seen when atrial contraction occurs at a time when the tricuspid valve is closed. Here the p wave is buried in the QRS complex, and large cannon waves can be seen. Irregular cannon waves of this type are also seen in complete atrioventricular block with atrioventricular dissociation. Regular cannon waves are seen in junctional tachycardia and in atrial tachycardia with rapid rates and a long P-R interval.

2. *Giant a wave:* The a wave is increased in force and amplitude in the presence of right ventricular hypertrophy. It is best seen as the "giant a wave" of pulmonary stenosis, which is a short, sharp, flicking wave occurring just before ventricular systole. A large a wave is also seen in pulmonary hypertension and in tricuspid valve disease with stenosis.

3. *Giant v wave:* A large v wave is seen in patients with tricuspid incompetence, especially when atrial fibrillation is present.

Tricuspid incompetence is seldom seen in patients with sinus rhythm, but when it occurs, a, x, v, and y peaks and troughs are present. The X descent is usually absent in patients with either tricuspid incompetence or pericardial constriction, and the Y descent may be the principal event in the venous pulse.

4. *Effect of inspiration:* Inspiration may stretch the tricuspid valve and make it incompetent, thus increasing the highest of the v wave and the depth of the y trough. Inspiration also increases the height of the a wave and enhances the X descent, in a patient in sinus rhythm. When right heart filling is severely impaired, inspiration causes a rise in venous pressure. This rise is known as Kussmaul's sign, and it is seen in pericardial constriction, and severe right heart failure. The overfilled right heart cannot accommodate the increased venous return associate with the inspiratory fall in intrathoracic pressure. The venous pressure therefore shows a rise with inspiration, instead of the normal fall. In tricuspid incompetence, it is the amplitude of the pulsations that tends to increase not the mean pressure, as in pericardial disease.

Arms

Brachial and radial pulses should be compared between the two arms, and they should also be compared with the femoral pulses. The fingers, nails, and palms should be examined for evidence of embolism. Femoral pulses normally come 80 msec earlier to radial artery but clinically they are felt simultaneously as human capacity to differentiate this small distance is lacking.

Fingers (Figs 2.9 to 2.15)

Clubbing of the fingers and nail beds is seen in cyanotic heart disease, in infective endocarditis, and in chronic lung disease, especially with cor pulmonale. Splinter hemorrhages in the nail beds should be sought as an indication of endocarditis, although it should be noted that similar findings might be seen in many normal people. Painful red, tender nodules in the pulp of the fingers or toes or on the palms or the soles are important evidence of embolism in infective endocarditis. They last for 4–5 days and gradually darken before fading and becoming painless. Such lesions seldom, if ever, suppurate. Other finger abnormalities associated with congenital heart disease include arachnodactyly, in which the fingers are long and spidery. This is seen in Marfan's syndrome and in some patients with atrial septal defect.

Lungs

Examination of the lungs in patients with heart disease focuses on the detection of pleural fluid and a search for rales/crepitations, especially at the base of the lungs posteriorly. Such findings reflect raised pulmonary venous pressure. Added sounds are noted when there is fluid in the alveoli, but the signs are not specific, and they may be absent in some cases of obvious pulmonary edema. They are often due to other causes. Pleural effusion due to heart failure is usually bilateral, in unilateral cases, it is commonest on the side on which the subject habitually lies. Evidence of collapse of the left lower lobe should be sought in patients with marked left atrial enlargement.

Some cardiac murmurs are heard well in the back. The best examples are the murmurs of coarctation of the aorta, increased bronchial collateral flow, and peripheral pulmonary artery stenosis; the last is often heard well in the axilla as well. Evidence of systemic collateral vessels in coarctation of the aorta is also well seen and felt in the back. Large, pulsating vessels can be detected near the angles of the scapulas. Edema of the lumbar region and sacrum is also sought while the physician examines the patient's back.

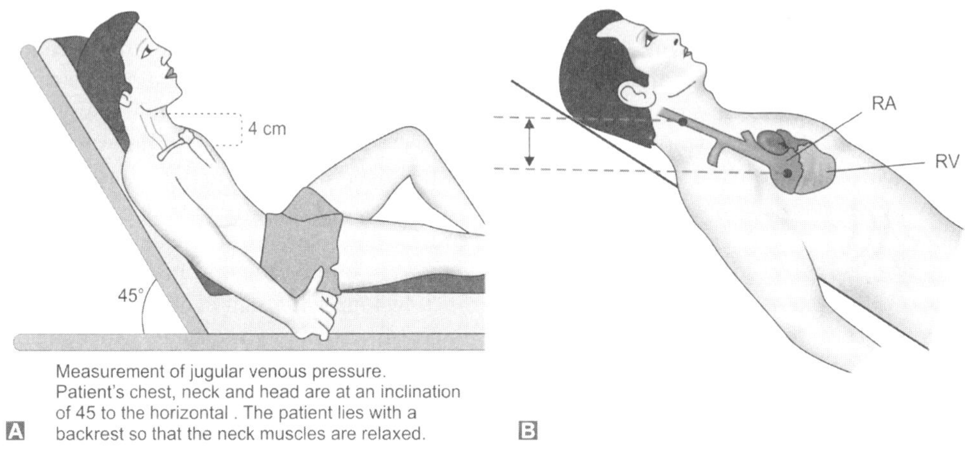

Figs 2.21A and B: Measurement of jugular venous pressure (JVP)

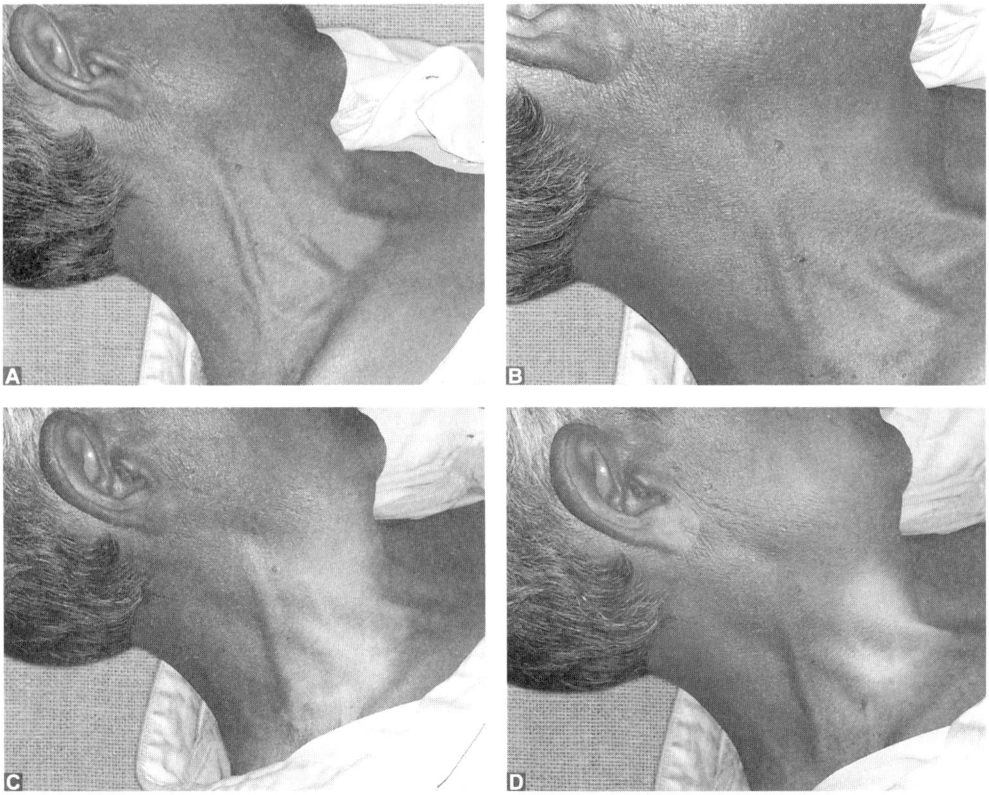

Figs 2.22A to D: Avoid easily visible external jugular vein

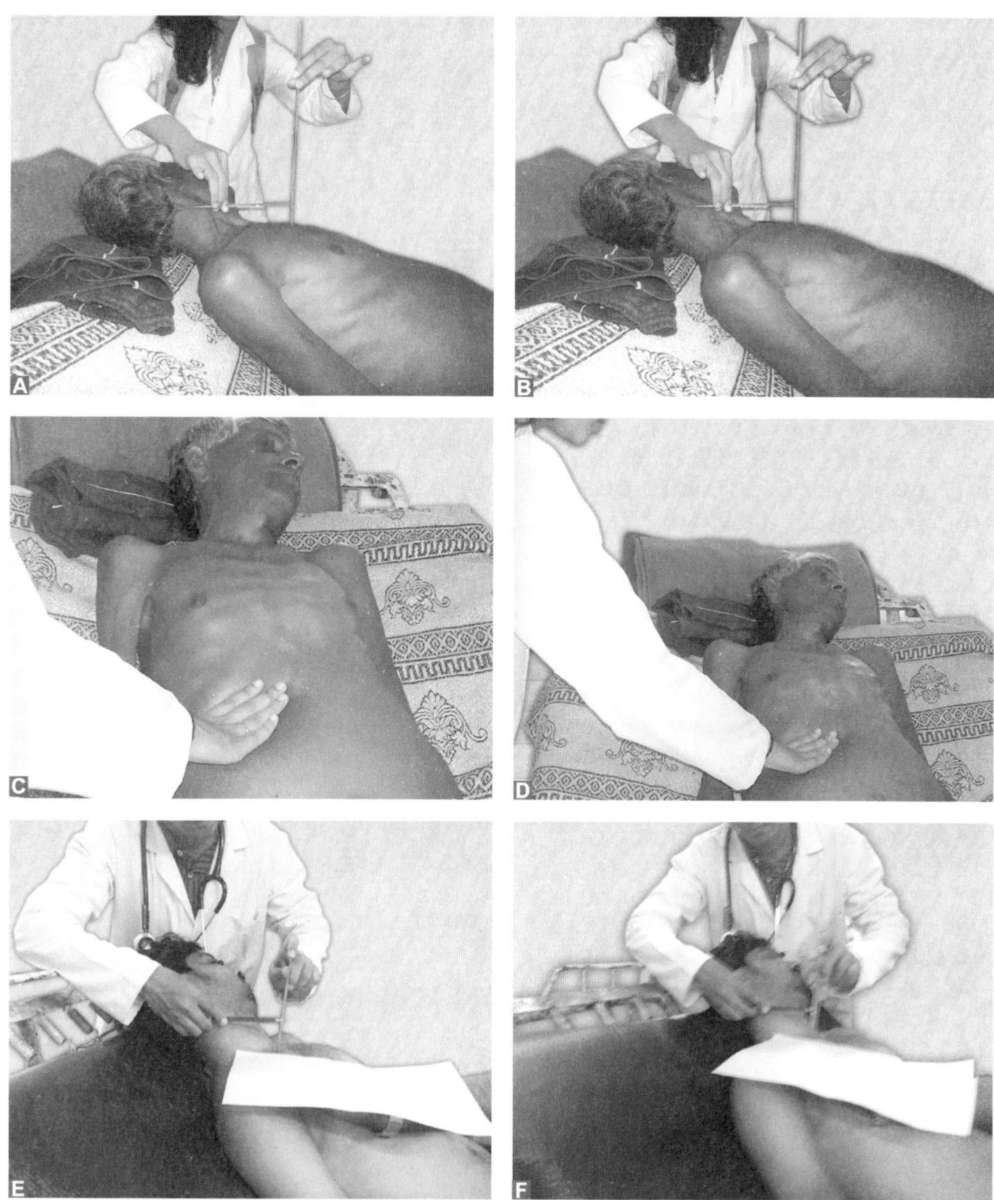

Figs 2.23A to F: Examination of jugular vein (Internal)

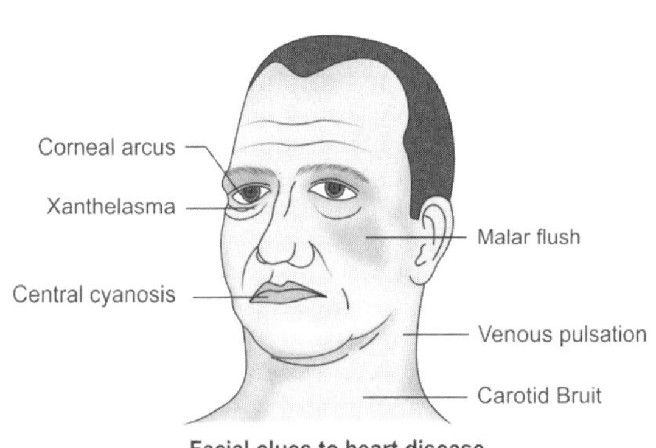

Fig. 2.24: Facial clues to heart disease

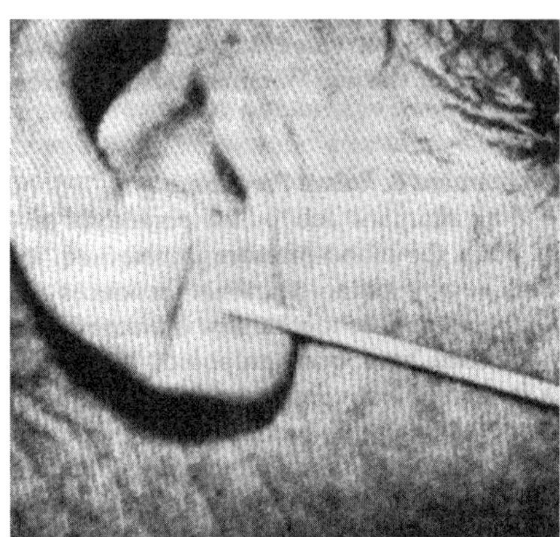

Fig. 2.25: Diagonal ear lobe create a sign of underlying CAD or atherosclerosis

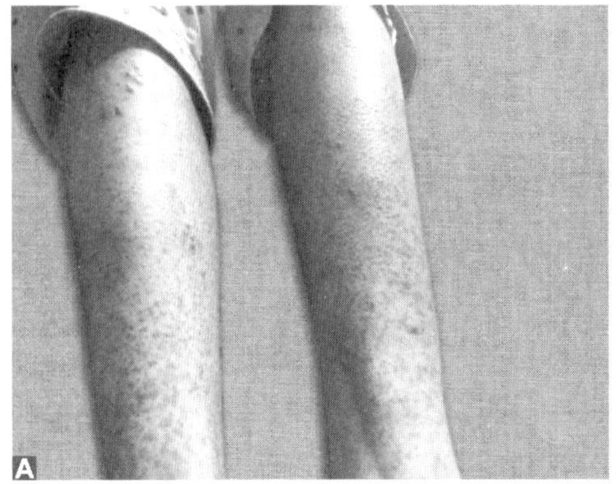

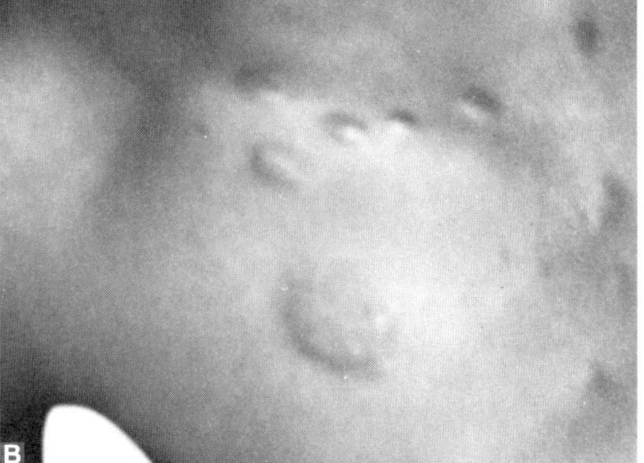

Figs 2.26A and B: Edema and pigmentation in legs

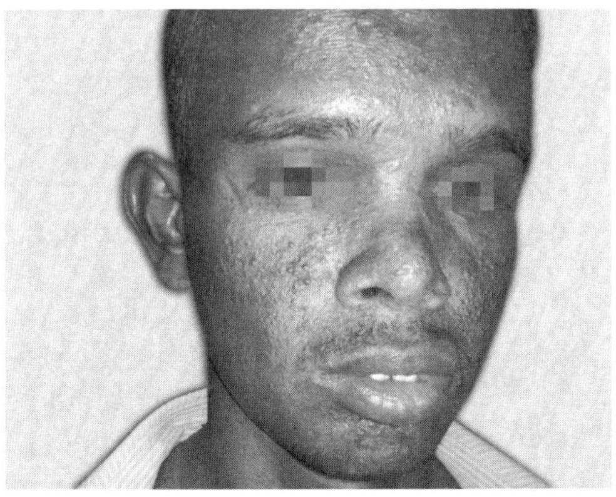

Fig. 2.27: Adenoma sebaceum

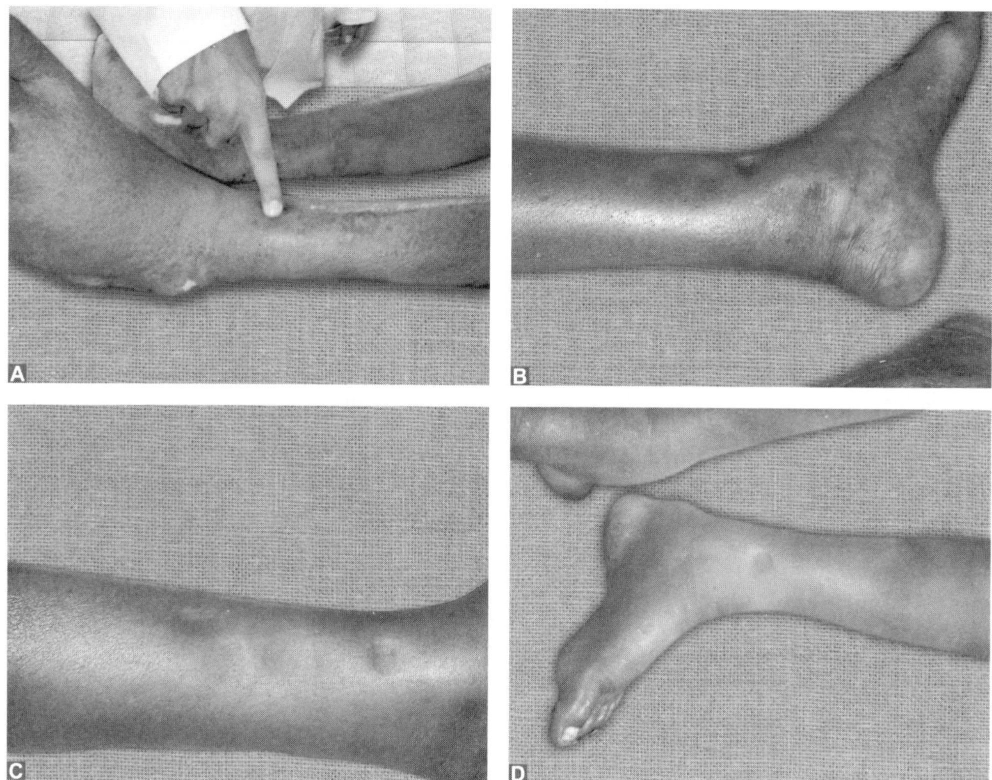

Figs 2.28A to D: Demonstratiion of pitting edema (Legs)

Abdomen (Figs 2.34 to 2.36)

In examining the abdomen, enlargement and tenderness of the liver and spleen should be sought as evidence of systemic venous congestion. The spleen may also be the site of a friction rub in infective endocarditis. Ascites and pitting edema of the ankles are also sought as evidence of congestive heart failure. Disproportionate ascites with minimal leg edema suggests pericardial constriction or prolonged diuretic therapy (Ascites Precox).

Lower Extremities (Fig. 2.26 and 2.28)

In examining the lower extremities, the physician palpates the femoral pulse, if its palpability is in question or if the patient is hypertensive, it is useful to look for delay between the radial and femoral pulse. Absence of femoral pulsation and inequality between the 2 sides may suggest embolic disease or aortic dissection. Calf tenderness and pain on dorsiflexion of the foot (Homans sign) are evidence of venous thrombosis. Clubbing of the toes is seen in cyanotic congenital heart disease, and differential cyanosis of the legs with clubbing, in the absence of similar findings in the arms, suggests patent ductus arteriosus with shunt reversal due to pulmonary hypertension. In addition to looking for edema of the sacrum, the examiner should check for edema in the flanks and medial aspects of the thighs in bedridden patients.

■ INSPECTION (FIG. 2.29)

Examination of the chest starts with inspection of the shape and movements of the thorax and a search for visible pulsations. Chest deformities such as kyphosis and scoliosis may cause heart disease, but in general, it is remarkable how a severe deformity can exist without causing cardiac embarrassment. Depressed sternum with pectus excavatum is obvious on inspection, and although it is often associated with benign heart murmurs, it is seldom of more than cosmetic importance. The left parasternal area sometimes bulges in patients who have had heart disease since early in life. Ventricular septal defect is the commonest lesion causing this sign.

Visible Pulsations

The cardiac impulse can sometimes be seen in normal subjects either in the area of the left nipple or in the epigastrium. Pulsation in the second or third left interspace over the right ventricular outflow tract can be seen in normal thin persons, but it can also suggest pulmonary hypertension or increased pulmonary blood flow. Pulsation to the right of the sternum is always abnormal, and when seen in the second or third interspace, it indicates aneurysmal dilatation of the ascending aorta.

Periodic Breathing

Abnormalities of respiratory rhythm should be noted during inspection of the chest. The commonest abnormality is periodic breathing. This can occur in normal subjects at high altitude and may also be seen after head injuries. When it is due to heart disease, the cycle of hyperventilation followed by hypoventilation and apnea with subsequent gradual increase of ventilation lasts 40–120 seconds. The phenomenon results from oscillation of the feedback control mechanisms regulating respiration. In a patient with severe ventricular failure, there is an abnormal lag between the timing of the neurologic stimulus to breathe and the arrival back at the control center in the brain of the humoral signal resulting from respiratory changes in blood gases following the breath. This lag is thought to play an important part in the mechanism of periodic breathing. Periodic breathing is usually referred to as Cheyne-Stokes breathing. In the classic description, apnea was present, but this feature is not necessarily a component. The length of the lung-to-brain circulation time determines the length of the period of one cycle. By following this measurement, the examination can note the progress of the patient's left ventricular failure. Periodic breathing is usually a manifestation of hyper rather than hypoventilation and is generally abolished by giving oxygen, CO_2, or aminophylline. It tends to occur at night when sensory input is low and to disappear when a mouthpiece and nose clip are used to obtain spirometric tracings. The level of ventilation can be deduced from the CO_2 level in the expired air, it is lowest when end tidal CO_2 is highest and vice versa. The respiratory rate varied during the cycle, which lasted about 45 seconds. Arterial oxygen saturation is out of phase with ventilation; arterial pressure tends to fall when ventilation is low and tends to rise with hyperpnea.

Palpation

Palpation of the chest is used to confirm the presence of pulsations that have been noted on inspection. The cardiac impulse is routinely sought and can be elicited by having the patient roll over to the left side. The examiner should note the nature of the impulse and distinguish between the feel of a large left ventricle and a right ventricle. The site where the impulse is felt is of primary importance in distinguishing the two impulses; in addition, the right ventricular impulse is more lifting than the left, is perceived as being further from the hand, and less readily moves the examining fingers (Figs 2.31A to D). The feel of a ventricle with a large stroke volume should be distinguished from the feel of a hypertrophied ventricle. Hypertrophy imparts a forceful thrust with relatively little movement of the examiner's hand, whereas increased stroke volume gives a more dynamic movement of greater amplitude. A "tapping" impulse is found in patients within mitral valve disease. This reflects the palpable vibrations of a loud first heart sound felt at the apex.

Apex Beat (Figs 2.30, 2.32 and 2.33)

It should not be confused with point of maximal impulse (PMI). The position of the apex beat should always be located by palpation. It is the point farthest downward and outward at which the cardiac impulse can be clearly felt. Before the determination of cardiac size by chest radiography became routine, the position of the apex beat in the absence of lung disease was the most important measure of heart size. Its position should be described in relation to the intercostal space and to the distance from the midline, the nipple, or this midclavicular, anterior axillary, or midaxillary lines. These are imaginary lines drawn vertically through various planes. Palpation of the base of the heart may detect an impulse caused by closure of the aortic or pulmonary valves or arising from an aneurysm. The findings should be interpreted in light of the patient's build. In meaning distance of apex beat from the midline tangential and not circumferential disease should be measured with important in obese

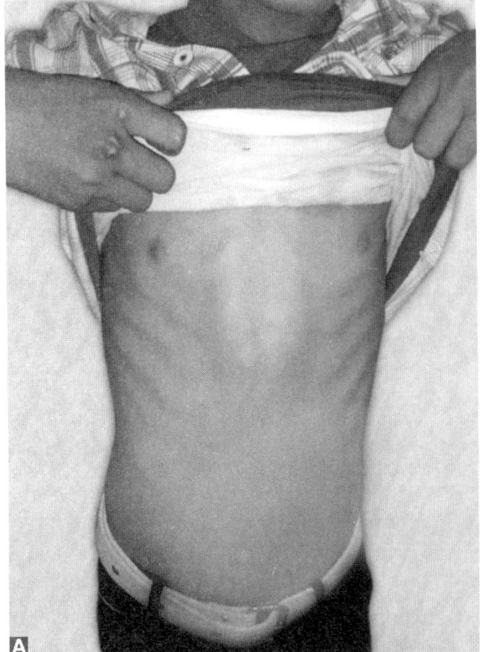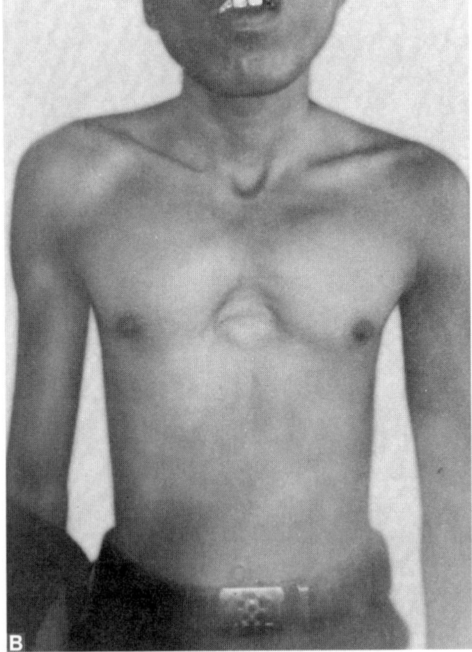

Figs 2.29A and B: Chest inspection

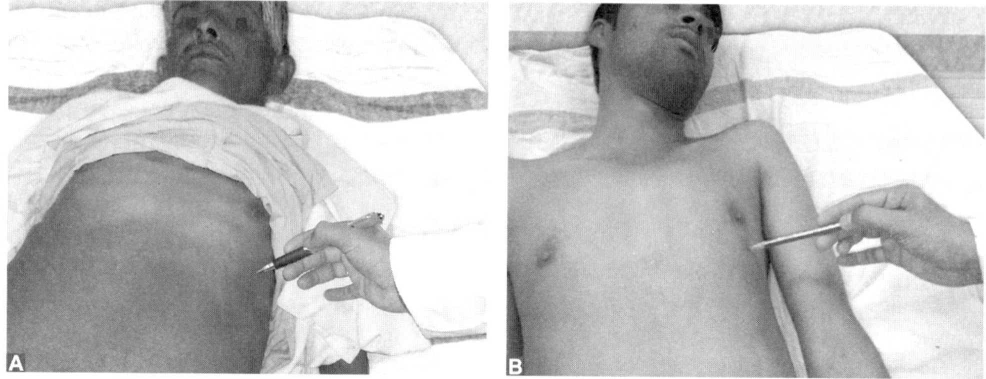

Figs 2.30A and B: Apex beat

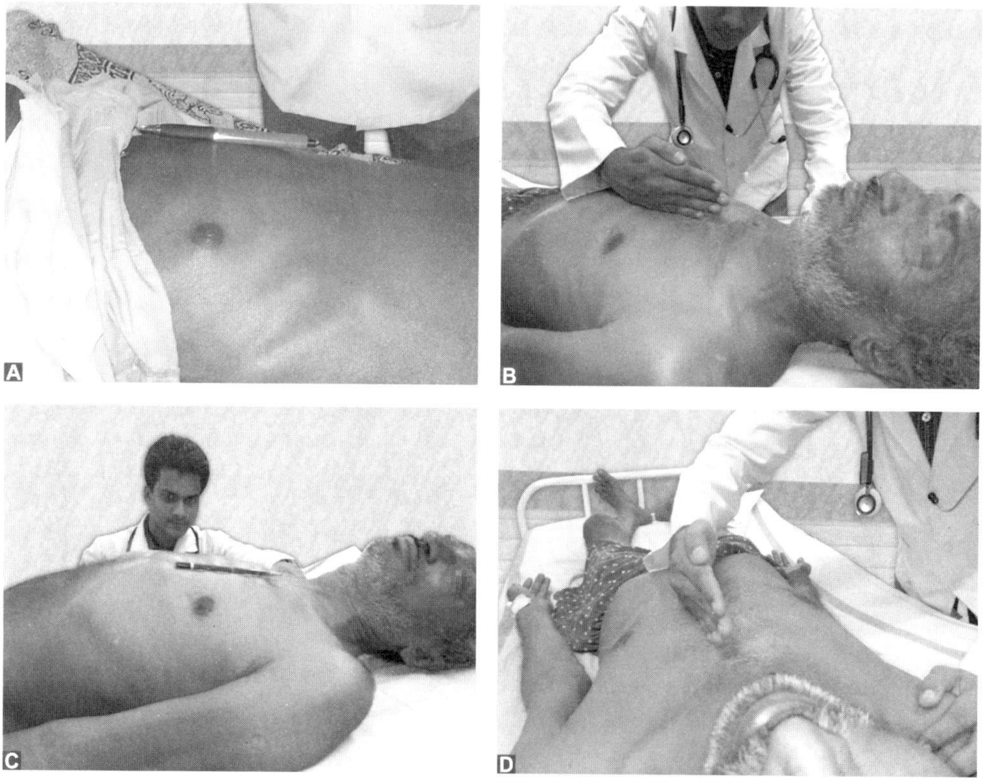

Figs 2.31A to D: Parasternal heave

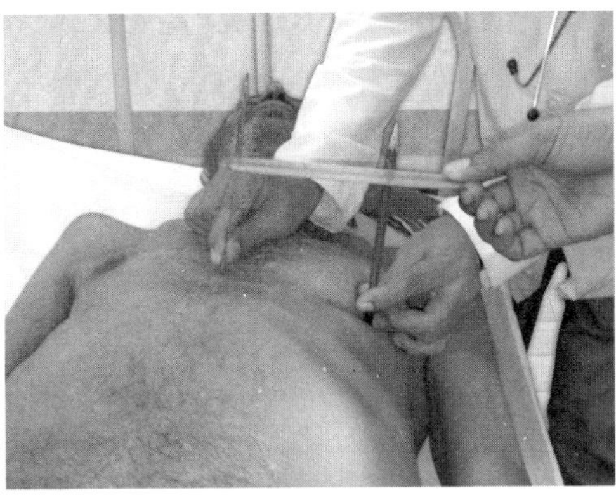

Fig. 2.32: Localization of apex—beat correct method tangential distance

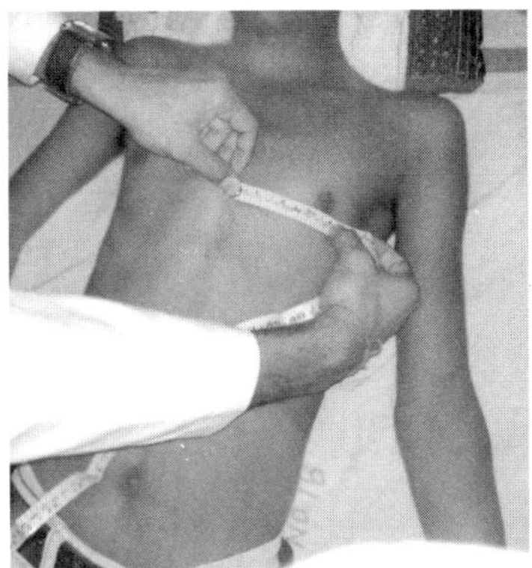

Fig. 2.33: Apex beat localization—incorrect method (Circumferential distance)

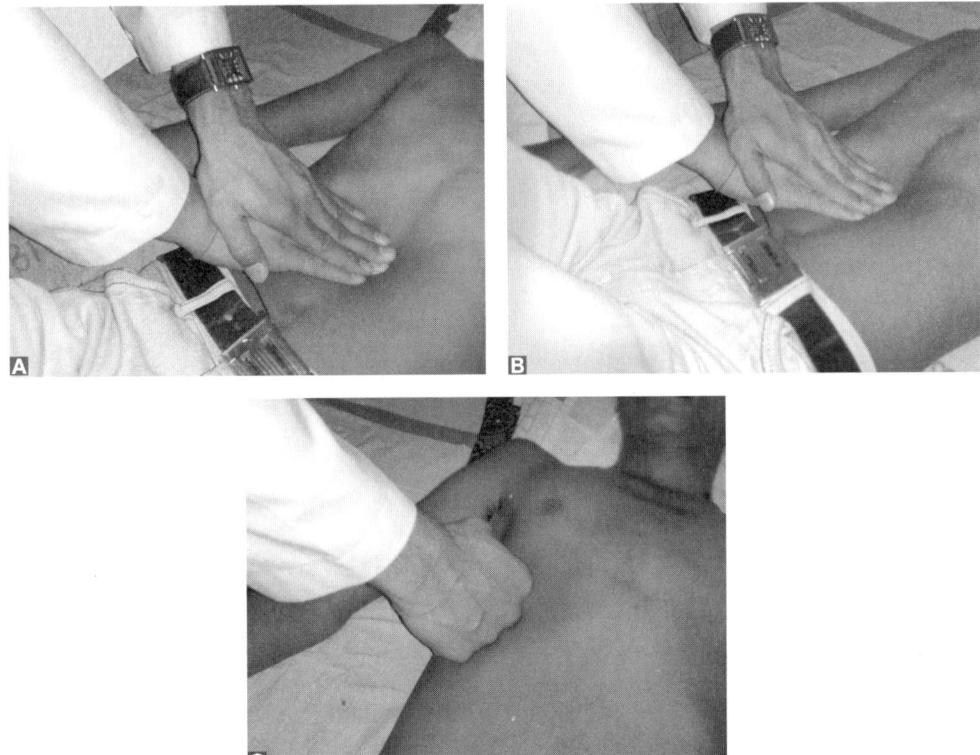

Figs 2.34A to C: Hepatic pulsation and palpation—hepatic pulsations when liver not enlarged

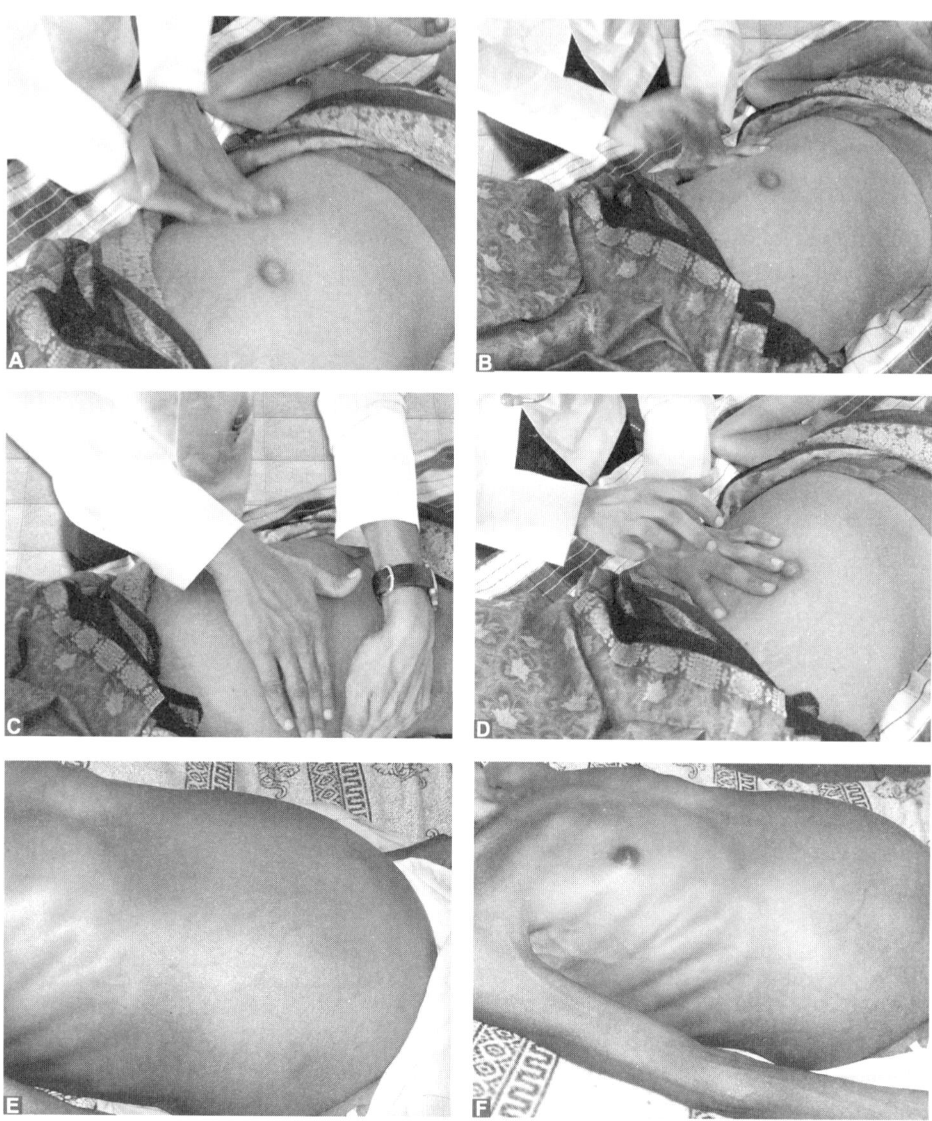

Figs 2.35A to F: Abdomen—ascites, hepatic palpation

present. Start from posterior axillary and more toward midline.

Thrills

The significance of palpable thrills is similar to that of cardiac murmurs and is discussed below (see Auscultation). Thrills are merely palpable, sustained high frequency vibrations associated with the same disturbances of flow that cause heart murmurs. A murmur that is associated with a thrill is likely to have an organic cause. Most sensitive part of hand free thrills is base of fingers joining with metacarpals.

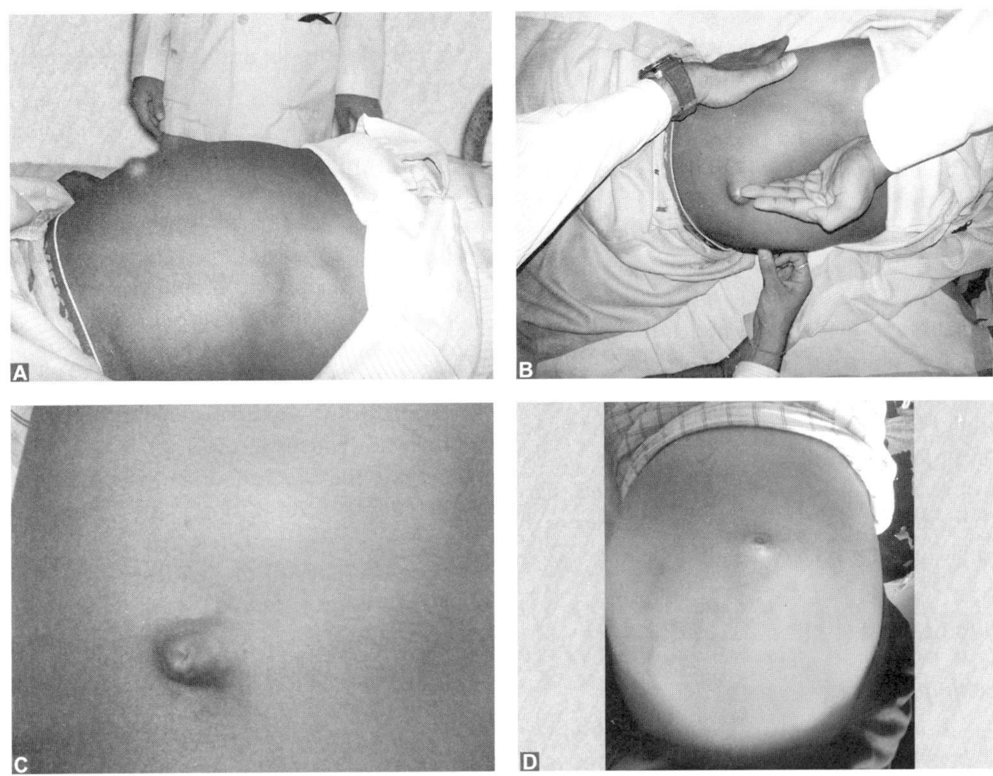

Figs 2.36A to D: Ascites

Palpable Impulses

Palpable impulses over the precordium must be interpreted in light of their associated findings, it is not always possible to be certain of their origin. In a patient with mitral incompetence, a substernal impulse may be due to systolic expansion of the left atrium rather than to right ventricular overactivity. It is also difficult to interpret epigastric pulsations. They may arise from the abdominal aorta or the right ventricle or be transmitted from the right atrium to an enlarged liver in tricuspid incompetence.

Using a pencil keeping it on chest and seeing it tangentially makes visible some otherwise invisible pulsations (Figs 2.31A to D Parasternal heare).

Paradoxical rocking impulses can sometimes be felt after myocardial infarction, especially when a left ventricular aneurysm is present. When the aneurysm involves the free ventricular wall, the outward motion of the aneurismal sac can sometimes be felt in early systole.

Palpable Gallops

The vibrations produced by loud third and fourth heart sounds can often be felt. If the sounds are of very low pitch, the gallop may be easier to appreciate on palpation than on auscultation. In most cases, in which a gallop is palpable, it is also audible. Sometimes these sounds can be made 'visible' by using a pencil held lightly over apex.

Percussion

Percussion of the heart has virtually lost its place in physical examination today because it is open to error and because the size of the heart is better determined by chest radiography. Before this method was routinely available, some confirmation of the estimate of heart size obtained by palpation was sought by percussion. Dullness to the right of the sternum was held to be evidence of pericardial effusion, and percussion of the left border was routinely advocated. Radiography has indicated that findings obtained by percussing the heart tend to be unreliable in all but the most skilled hands. However, the only unambiguous physical sign of pericardial effusion is the demonstration of cardiac dullness outside the apex beat.

Auscultation (Figs 2.37 and 2.46)

Technique

Auscultation of the heart is performed with a properly fitting stethoscope that uses either an open bell or a closed diaphragm as the means of coupling the examiner's ear to the patient's chest. The diaphragm transmits more sound and is better for listening to high-pitched sounds (such as the second heart sound) and murmurs. The bell is better for low-pitched noises, and variation of the pressure of the bell on the skin can be used to alter the intensity of the sounds and murmurs heard. Auscultation focuses more on the timing of events within the cardiac cycle than on their intensity or the site at which they are heard well. Experienced physicians move the chest piece of the stethoscope to sites where they can best hear specific sounds. They do not restrict their examination to the classic 'valvular' areas described in older textbooks. They also do not draw conclusions about the origin of events from the site at which they hear sounds and murmurs. The information obtained by auscultation must be integrated with that already obtained by inspection and palpation. Do not press bell of stethoscope too hard on chest wall otherwise underlying skin may stretch and start acting as diaphragm and low frequencies will be dismissed.

Heart Sounds (Figs 2.45A to D)

First and second heart sounds are normally audible, and an early (diastolic gallop) third sound is often present in children and young adults. In addition, a fourth (atrial) sound can sometimes be recorded by phonocardiography.

A. *First Heart Sound:* The first heart sound (S1) is attributed to closure of the mitral and tricuspid valves at the start of ventricular systole. The two components can sometimes be clearly distinguished, and although the right atrial and right ventricular contractions precede those of the left, the mitral valve closes before the tricuspid, and the first component of the first heart sound is mitral in origin. The position of the valve leaflets at the time of the start of systole influences the loudness of the first sound. In general, the first heart sound is louder, longer, and lower pitched than the second heart sound at the apex. In normal resting subjects, the atrioventricular valve leaflets have drifted into on almost closed position by the time systole starts, because diastolic flow is more or less complete by late diastole. Atrial contraction tends to reopen the valves. Consequently, the length of the P-R interval affects the loudness of the first sound. When flow across an atrioventricular valve is increased, for any reason or lasts longer than normally, the valve tends to shut from a more open position and produces more noise. The situation is similar to that encountered in closing an open door; the wider the door stands open before it is slammed shut, the louder the resulting noise. Thus, a loud first sound is heard in patients who are exercising, in patients with mitral stenosis in whom flow lasts throughout the whole of diastole, and in patients with left-to-right shunts and increased atrioventricular flow, e.g. atrial septal defect. In complete atrioventricular block in which the P-R interval varies, the loudness of the first sound varies, being loudest when the P-R interval is slightly shortened to about 0.1 second.

B. *Second Heart Sound:* The second heart sound (S2) is due to closure of the semilunar valves and normally consists of 2 components. The earlier component is normal aortic in origin; the later one arises from the pulmonary valve (P2). The location at which the second heart sound is best heard varies. It is normally heard well at the base and is usually louder than the first sound in that area. It is sometimes necessary to listen at the apex or even in the epigastrium.

1. **Splitting of the second heart sound:** Right and left ventricular stroke volumes vary reciprocally with quiet respiration when there is adequate venous return. Inspiration favors right ventricular output, and expiration favors left ventricular output. Thus, in normal subjects resting quietly and breathing easily, the time of pulmonary valve closure with inspiration can be shown to more later in the cardiac cycle by 0.02–0.04 see. Increased filling of the right heart is associated with a more negative pressure within the thorax during inspiration, which increases right ventricular output in accordance with the Frank-Starling mechanism. The extra output has a longer ejection time; consequently, the pulmonary valve closure sound is delayed. The opposite occurs with aortic valve closure during expiration, but the magnitude of the changes is less. Thus, although both the aortic and pulmonary components of the second heart sound move, the pulmonary component moves more. The net effect is that the interval between the two components of the second sound increases with inspiration and then decreases until the interval between the

two sounds is not appreciable during expiration. The process is conventionally referred to as physiologic splitting of the second heart sound. When right ventricular systole is prolonged because of right bundle branch block, pulmonary valve closure is delayed. In this case, both the first and the second heart sounds tend to be split throughout the cardiac cycle, with the split widening further with inspiration. When right ventricular stroke volume is increased and venous return is high, as in atrial septal defect with large pulmonary blood flow, respiration has relatively little effect on right ventricular output. In this case, pulmonary valve closure is greatly delayed and the second sound is widely split, respiration has no effect, and the split is 'fixed' even during expiration. Splitting of the second heart sound is usually found in atrial septal defect with left-to-right shunt, but the finding of a fixed split is indicative of significant left-to-right shunt. If the venous return is reduced when the patient stands up, the splitting of the second sound will become more normal, becoming either movable with respiration or less widely split.

2. **Paradoxical splitting of the second sound:** When left ventricular contraction is prolonged (e.g. poor contractility, aortic stenosis), aortic valve closure is delayed and occurs after pulmonary closure. Aortic valve closure can be identified by timing it against the dicrotic notch of the carotid artery tracing. In paradoxical splitting, aortic and pulmonary valve closure sounds coincide towards the end of inspiration and splitting is greatest during expiration. This is also referred to as "reversed" splitting of the second sound and is found in patients with left bundle branch block, in aortic stenosis, and in any other condition that greatly overloads the left ventricle. The

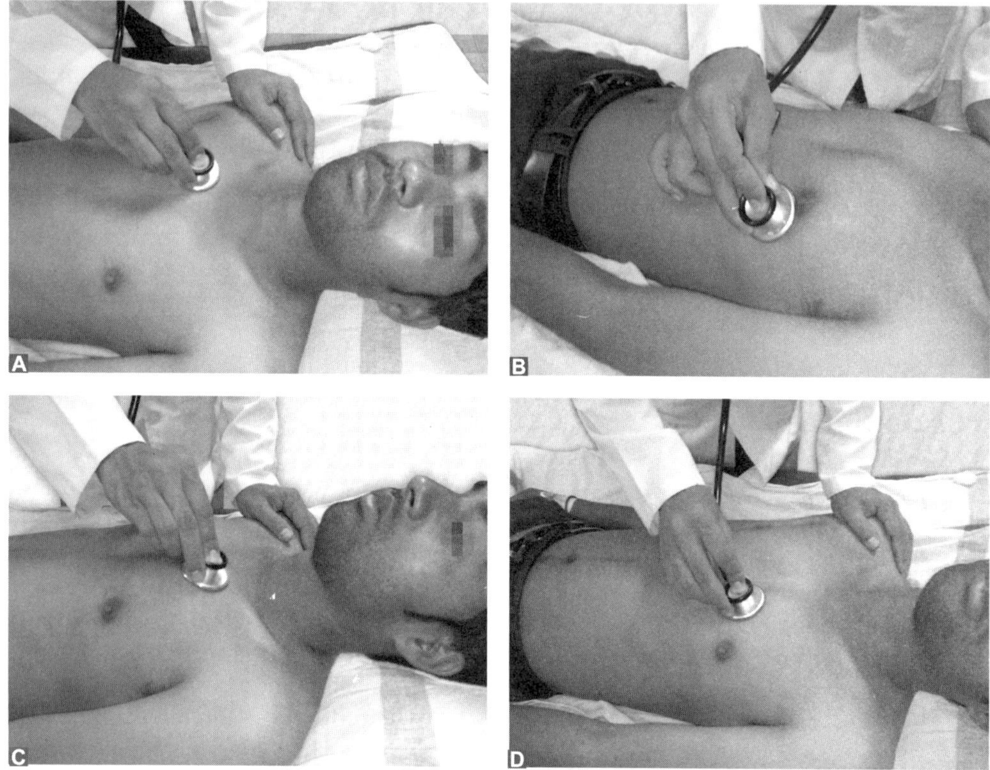

Figs 2.37A to D: Auscultation of heart in different ausculatory area, (A) Aortic areas; (B) Mitral area; (C) Pulmonary area; (D) Tricuspid area

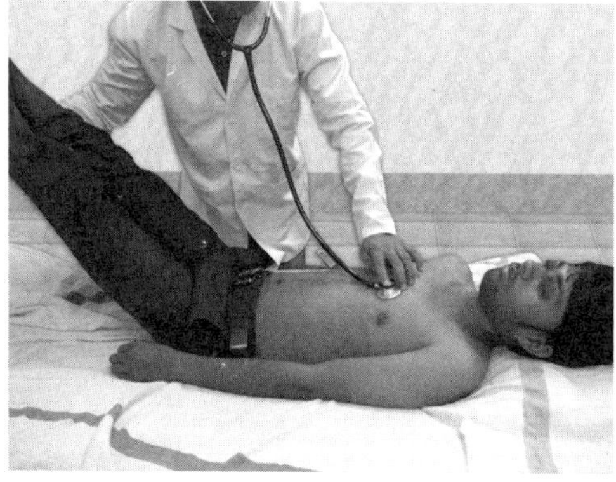

Fig. 2.38: Posing leg raising test to accentuate tricuspid regurgitation murmur (Carvallo's sign)

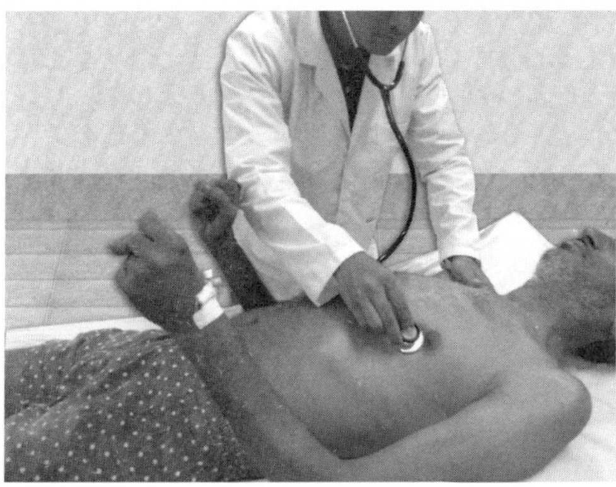

Fig. 2.39: Mitral area auscultation

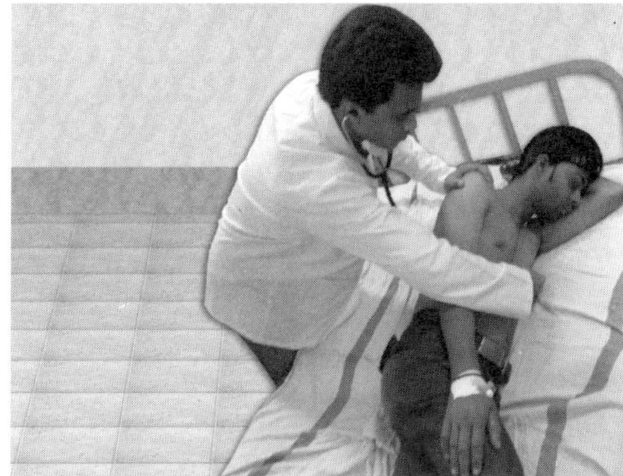

Fig. 2.40: Auscultation in left lateral position (mitral area)

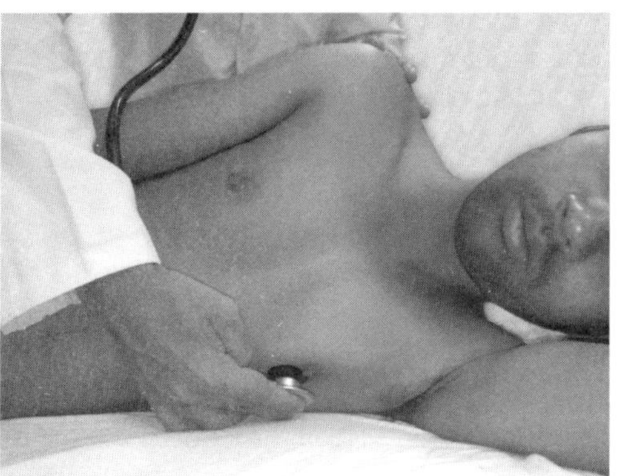

Fig. 2.41: Auscultation for murmur of mitral stenosis using bell of stethoscope chest piece

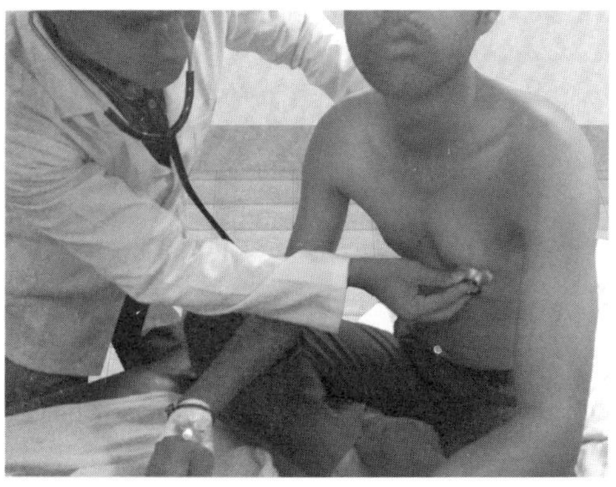

Fig. 2.42: Auscultation in sitting position

effect of respiration on the second heart sound in paradoxical splitting is aortic valve closure tends to be delayed and diminished in aortic stenosis and may be absent when the lesion is severe. The reason for this is not known. In systemic hypertension, the aortic valve closure sound is not only loud but also clear and ringing.

C. **Third Heart Sound:** The third heart sound (S3) is associated with ventricular filling. It is not clear why it is normally present in young persons and disappears with age. An audible third heart sound is also found when there is an abnormally large diastolic flow into a normal ventricle, or a normal flow into an abnormal ventricle. The former occurs in patients with left-to-right shunt and also occurs in mitral or tricuspid incompetence. The latter is seen in patients with right or, more commonly, left ventricular disease. The third heart sound is a dull, low-pitched, localized sound occurring about 0.12–0.16 sec after the second sound. If the sound arises from the right heart, it increases in intensity during inspiration and is heard at the lower

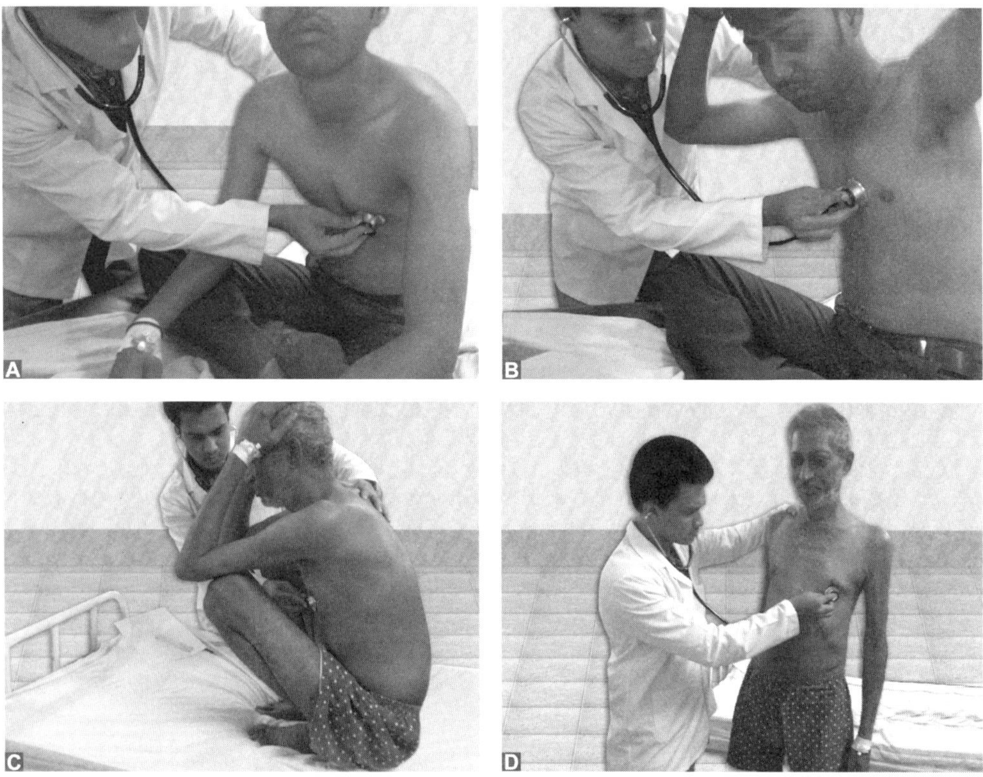

Figs 2.43A to D: Auscultation of heart in different position, (A) Sitting; (B) Sitting with arms above head (AR); (C) Squatting position; (D) Auscultation in standing position

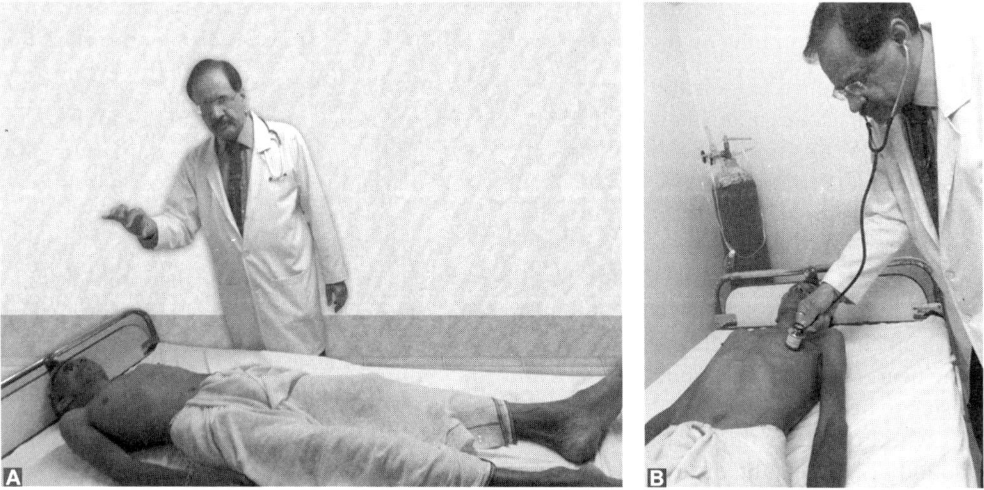

Figs 2.44A and B: Objective grading of intensity of heart sounds and murmur

sterna edge. Conversely, a left sided third sound increases on expiration.

D. **Fourth Heart Sound:** The fourth heart sound (S4) results from atrial contraction and is thought to be a filling sound arising within the ventricle. Although it can often be recorded by phonocardiography, it is not normally audible. A fourth heart sound is heard shortly before the first heart sound in any condition in which the force of either the right or the left atrial contraction is increased. This means that atrial sounds are heard in conditions in which the ventricle is working against high pressure and the atria are contracting against increased resistance. Thus, pulmonary or aortic stenosis and pulmonary or systemic hypertension are the commonest causes of a fourth heart sound. A fourth heart sound is also often audible during an episode of angina pectoris. Here, too, the ventricular compliance is reduced, and the left atrium contracts against increased resistance. Right and left atrial sounds can often be distinguished on the basis of their response to respiration and the site where they are most clearly heard.

E. **Gallop Rhythm:** When a third or a fourth heart sound is present, the extra heart sounds give rise to a gallop, or triple, rhythm. When the extra sound is presystolic, it is difficult to distinguish the rhythm from that of a split first sound or even an ejection click following the first sound. The presystolic gallop is said to have the cadence of the word "Tennessee," whereas diastolic gallop has been likened to "Kentucky". In some cases, both third and fourth heart sounds can be heard. If the heart rate is rapid—about 120/min the third and fourth sounds may be superimposed, giving rise to "summation" gallop. In this case, two inaudible sounds may combine to give an audible sound. It is possible to slow the heart rate by carotid sinus massage and listen to hear whether the gallop disappears or whether either the third or the fourth sound or both can be distinguished, which causes a quadruple rhythm. A prominent

filling sound is also heard in patients with impaired ventricular filling in pericardial constriction. This can be as loud a sound as the second heart sound and is sometimes called a "pericardial knock". It is thought to be caused by the sudden cessation of right ventricular filling.

F. **Opening Snap:** The opening snap of the atrioventricular valve heard in patients with rheumatic valvular disease is also considered as a heart sound. It is heard 0.06–0.12 second after the second heart sound and it may be the loudest and most widely heard sound in the cardiac cycle and is heard best in the third or fourth left interspace in most cases.

G. **Systolic Clicks:** Extra intracardiac sounds are also heard during systole. These, like the opening snap, arise from valves. The commonest is the systolic ejection click, which can arise from either the aortic or the pulmonary valve. The click occurs early in systole, about 0.02 second after the first sound. It usually ushers in a systolic ejection murmur. Ejection clicks commonly occur when dilatation of the great vessel (aorta or pulmonary artery) with which they are associated is combined with normal or increased flow through the vessel. They are louder during expiration, when the walls of the vessel are less taut, because the intrathoracic pressure is less negative. Ejection clicks are sometimes heard in normal subjects but are most common in patients with insignificant or mild stenosis of the associated valve. A different variety of systolic click is heard in patients with insignificant mitral incompetence. The clicks, which may be multiple, occur in mid or even late systole and may precede, follow, or accompany the late systolic murmur heard in this lesion (click murmur syndrome). In some cases, the click occurs without any murmur. The basic lesion is prolapse of the mitral valve cusp, and although the sound is thought to originate in the valve, the exact mechanism of its production is not known.

Heart Murmurs (Figs 2.45A to D)

Cardiac murmurs are thought to result from disturbances of normal blood flow patterns in the heart and great vessels. They are classified on the basis of their timing as systolic diastolic, and continuous murmurs.

A. **Systolic Murmurs:** Systolic murmurs are generally less significant than diastolic murmurs and may occur in patients in whom no evidence of heart disease can be found.

1. *Ejection murmurs:* An abnormally large flow through a normal valve may cause a systolic murmur, which is ejection in timing. An ejection murmur begins when flow starts in one of the great vessels and finishes before the time of valve closure. It thus starts after the first heart sound and ends before the second heart sound. Systolic ejection murmurs can be heard in high output states such as anemia, pregnancy, or thyrotoxicosis and also in patients with dilated aortic root due to atherosclerosis, hypertension, syphilis, or other forms of aortitis. They occur when there is a high stroke volume, as in complete atrioventricular block with bradycardia. Increased flow through the pulmonary valve occurs in patients with left-to-right shunts, especially in atrial septal defect, and a systolic ejection murmur is virtually always found in such conditions.

   The most important causes of systolic ejection murmurs are aortic and pulmonary stenoses at a valvular level. The intensity and duration of such murmurs vary with the severity of the stenosis and with the stroke volume. When the stroke volume is low, the murmur may be of low intensity, and it does not last as long as it does when there is normal flow. Because a systolic ejection murmur can also occur when the stenosis is mild and the valve is merely thickened, it is unwise to base any assessment of the severity of the stenosis on the intensity of the murmur.

2. *Pansystolic murmurs:* Pansystolic (holosystolic) murmurs start with the first sound and continue up to the second sound. They are commonly due to incompetence of the mitral or tricuspid valve. The valve leaks throughout systole, and the relatively high pressure difference across the valve accounts for the murmur. The murmur is high-pitched and more musical (or purer tone) than an ejection murmur. A similar murmur is heard when there is flow across a ventricular septal defect with a large pressure difference between the two ventricles.

3. *Late systolic murmurs:* Mitral incompetence can also result in a late systolic murmur that increases in intensity up to the second sound. This murmur has a peculiar quality, and inexperienced observes may find it difficult to time. Once recognized, it is never forgotten. This late systolic murmur may become pansystolic when the degree of incompetence increases, e.g. when peripheral resistance is increased during the overshoot that occurs following Valsalva's maneuver.

4. *Other systolic murmurs:* Although in theory it is easy to classify murmurs as ejection or pansystolic, it may be difficult to make this distinction in practice. In some cases, the murmur exhibits features of both varieties, and it varies in timing at different sites. In infundibular stenosis involving the outflow tract of the right ventricle or in hypertrophic obstructive cardiomyopathy, which produces a rather similar lesion in the left ventricle, there is usually a harsh murmur, which lasts throughout systole but peaks in intensity in the middle of systole, when flow is greatest. Similarly, when pulmonary stenosis

and ventricular septal defect coexist, the murmur has characteristics of both pansystolic and ejection murmurs.

A special type of systolic murmur may occur in coarctation of the aorta or peripheral pulmonary arterial stenosis. In these conditions, there may be a murmur late in systole owing to the late peaking of flow across the narrowing in the vessel. In coarctation, there may also be a systolic murmur, which lasts longer and is due to flow through collateral vessels in the chest wall which have developed in response to the lesion. This murmur is similar to that of bronchial collateral flow, which is heard in patients who have markedly reduced flow to the lungs via the pulmonary artery, as in pulmonary atresia. This systolic murmur also resembles the bruit heard over an arteriovenous fistula or over an extremely active toxic goiter. Systolic bruits are also heard over stenotic lesions in peripheral vessels. Carotid arterial and renal arterial stenotic lesions are the most important examples. These murmurs can be systolic or diastolic in timing and are ejection in character. They tend to occur late in the cardiac cycle.

B. Diastolic Murmurs: Diastolic murmurs are at most always due to significant lesions, although they can rarely occur in severe anemia. They are either immediate, caused by incompetence of the aortic or pulmonary valve, or delayed, caused by actual or relative mitral or tricuspid stenosis. A special form of diastolic murmur that is commonest in mitral stenosis is the atrial systolic, or presystolic, murmur.

1. *Immediate (early diastolic) murmurs:* Immediate, or early, diastolic murmurs start immediately after the time of closure of the appropriate valve. They decrease in intensity during diastole and are high pitched and difficult to hear. They are heard best using the diaphragm of the stethoscope, with the subject sitting up and leaning forward and the breath held in expiration. These murmurs are heard on either side of the sternum in the third, fourth, and fifth interspaces. Their duration is roughly related to the severity of the valvular lesion. Similar murmurs are heard when there is diastolic flow from the aorta into any low pressure chamber, e.g. the right ventricle or an atrium.

2. *Delayed (middiastolic) murmurs:* The delayed or middiastolic, murmur does not start until the ventricular pressure has fallen below the level of the atrial pressure. There is thus a sound-free interval between the second heart sound and the start of the murmur. The murmur is low pitched and rumbling, and its duration is related to the severity of the stenosis and the size of the stroke volume. Mitral stenosis is the commonest cause of such a murmur; patent ductus arteriosus and ventricular septal defect on the left side and atrial septal defect and tricuspid stenosis on the right side are other causes. Pure tricuspid stenosis is rare, but mixed incompetence and stenosis does occasionally give rise to a delayed diastolic murmur. The right-sided murmurs increase with inspiration and are heard near the sternum. The left-sided murmurs are best heard with the patient lying in the left lateral position and the stethoscope applied directly over the point of maximal cardiac impulse.

3. *Presystolic murmurs:* Presystolic accentuation of a delayed diastolic murmur is characteristics of mitral stenosis. In some cases, the presystolic murmur is all that can be heard at rest with the patient supine. The delayed diastolic murmur is often elicited by having the patient exercise and then lie on the left side. Presystolic accentuation of a murmur is also

encountered in patients with severe aortic incompetence (Austin Flint murmur). The aortic cusp of the mitral valve tends to caught between the two streams of blood during diastole. One stream flowing from the aorta through the leaking valve encounters another from the left atrium during diastolic ventricular filling. The valve leaflet tends to vibrate in the two streams and cause what Austin Flint described as a blubbering murmur. This murmur may appear or become louder at the time of atrial systole and thus be confused with the murmur of mitral stenosis. In practice, the two lesions mitral stenosis and aortic incompetence are readily distinguished, and it is only when the lesions are thought to coexist that difficulties in diagnosis arise.

4. *Continuous murmurs:* Continuous murmurs arise when there is a pressure difference between two communicating vessels or chambers at all times in the cardiac cycle. The commonest example is that found in patent ductus arteriosus with left-to-night shunt. This lesion gives rise to a continuous 'machinery' murmur. The characteristic feature of the murmur is that it is loudest at the time of the second heart sound. At this time, right ventricular ejection is coming to an end and pulmonary arterial pressure is falling while aortic pressure is remaining high. Similar continuous murmurs are heard with aortopulmonary fistulas and after surgical creation of a shunt for the relief of tetralogy of Fallot (Blaock's operation).

C. **Differential Diagnosis:** Murmurs that come close to being continuous can be readily confused with the 'machinery' murmur, if their relationship to the second heart sound is not taken into account. In mixed aortic stenosis and incompetence, a to-and-fro systolic and diastolic murmur can appear almost continuous. There is, however, a gap at the time of the second heart sound. Similarly, in patients with ventricular septal defect and aortic incompetence, the murmur may appear continuous. Coronary arteriovenous fistula and anomalous drainage of a coronary vessel into the pulmonary artery also give continuous murmurs, and in cases of rupture of a sinus of Valsalva aneurysm into a chamber with a lower pressure, the murmur is continuous or near continuous. The murmur of a patent ductus may only be heard high in the left chest below the left clavicle. In some patients, it may be confused with a venous hum. This is a sound that may be continuous and results from partial occlusion of a large vein. Such a bruit is abolished by pressure over the root of the neck or by a change in the patient's position. The hum is never loudest at the time of the second heart sound.

D. **Factors Influencing Murmurs:** The interpretation of the origin of murmurs can be assisted by determining the direction of transmission of the murmur. The stethoscope is moved over various areas of the precordium to determine where the murmur can still be heard. Murmurs arising from the mitral valve are transmitted toward the axilla. Aortic and pulmonary diastolic murmurs are transmitted down the sides of the sternum. Aortic stenotic murmurs are usually but not always transmitted into the neck. The information obtained from determining the direction of transmission of murmurs is only of secondary value, however. The tendency for right-sided murmurs to be accentuated with inspiration is of more significance than any tendency for a left-sided murmur to be louder during expiration. All intracardiac sounds tend to become less loud with inspiration simply because the stethoscope moves farther away from the origin of the sound and because lung tissue is likely to be interposed and decrease the sound transmission. Thus, exaggeration of a murmur by inspiration is of greater significance than an increase with expiration.

E. **Effects of Drugs and Valsalva's Maneuver:** Several simple devices and pharmacologic maneuvers have been advocated as aids in interpreting the origin of murmurs. Listening during the period of strain in Valsalva's maneuver or during the overshoot after release of the strain and determining the effect of amyl nitrite inhalation are perhaps the most popular methods. Right sided murmurs disappear or diminish early during the strain and return early after release of pressure in Valsalva's maneuver. The increase in arterial pressure during the period of overshoot tends to accentuate the murmur of mitral incompetence and decrease the intensity of murmurs in aortic stenosis and hypertrophic obstructive disease. Similar results can be obtained with the use of phenylephrine infusion to raise the systemic arterial pressure. Amyl nitrite reduces systemic resistance and thus accentuates the murmurs of aortic stenosis and obstructive cardiomyopathy and decreases the murmur of mitral incompetence.

Pericardial Friction Rubs

Pericardial friction rubs are heard over the precordium as harsh, grating sounds related to the cardiac cycle and having a systolic component. When they have several components—most typically they have three. It may be difficult to distinguish them from murmurs. They tend to vary with time, posture, and the phase of respiration. Their intensity tends to vary with the degree of pressure of the bell of the stethoscope on the chest and they sound superficial, like the noise of hair rubbing against the diaphragm of the stethoscope.

INTEGRATION OF CARDIAC PHYSICAL FINDINGS

The findings on inspection, palpation, and auscultation must all be integrated to form an overall opinion of the likely clinical diagnosis. The heart sounds, clicks, snaps, and murmurs described from the basis of the classic physical findings seen in cardiac lesions.

Some Objective Gradings in Cardiology Palpation and Auscultation

Many physical signs in cardiology physical examination are traditionally marred by variations in reporting due to subjective variations between different physicians' experience, skills and at time physical acuity. Sometimes it is difficult to convey to other fellow physician about exact loudness of heart sounds, murmurs, intensity of respiratory sounds. Similarly force of parasternal leave, apex beat force and duration are also subject to marked various in reporting these events. Moreover, comparing these physical signs in the same patient after few days or weeks may also be difficult due to lack of objective grading. Here I have tried to objective some cardiac events like duration and force of apex beat, intensity of heart sounds and murmurs.

Intensity of heart murmurs and heart sounds: Heart sounds and murmurs are variably reported by different physicians as loud, very loud, soft or faint or very faint. These objectives may mean different to different doctors even if there are having normal hearing acuity, matters may be worse is their heaving abilities are also different. Levine long time back tried to grade intensity of murmurs:

Grade 1: A faint murmur heart with difficulty and with concentration in a quiet room by an experienced physician.

Grade 2: An easily heard murmur.

Grade 3: A loud murmurs without thrill.

Grade 4: A loud murmur with thrill.

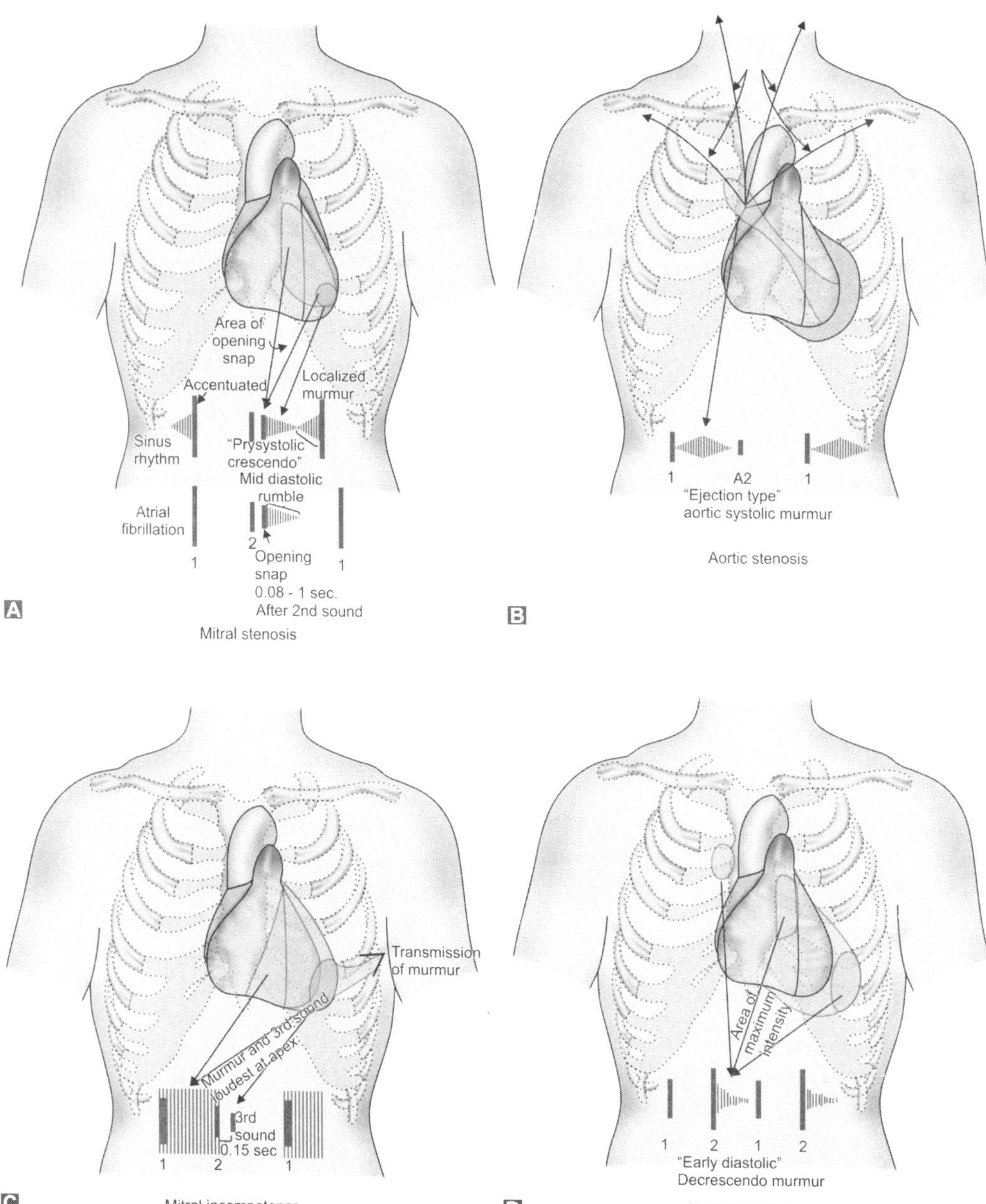

Figs 2.45A to D: Description of heart sound and murmurs in various valvular disease

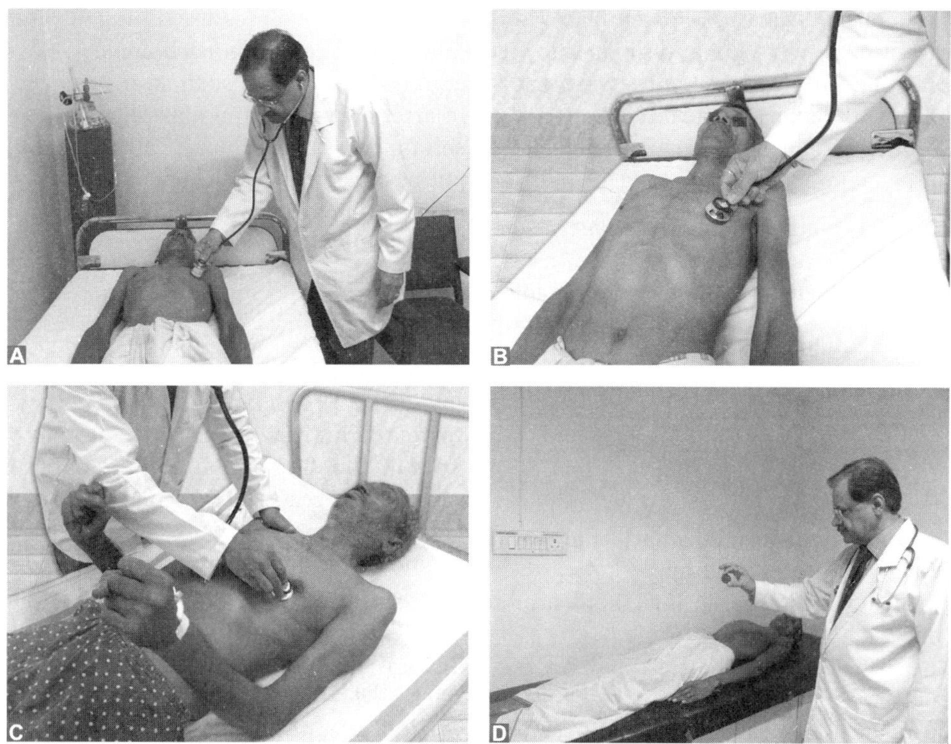

Figs 2.46A to D: Objective grading of intensity of heart murmurs and heart sounds using standardized discs
(*Source:* The lancet measurement of intetisity of heart sounds and murmurs Sharma RS, P 612, 19 sept 1981)

Grade 5: A very loud murmur heard with edge of stethoscope on chest wall.

Grade 6: A very loud murmur heard with stethoscope chest piece away from chest wall

However, this grading is also affected by subjective variations in skill and hearing power. Murmur easily heard by senior cardiologist may be easily underestimated or not heard easily by a novice/intern. Author (Dr RSS) put forward a more objective grading of murmur and heart sound which was published in 'The Lancet". It is as follows: Murmur and heart sounds are heard in usual way and then standardized plastic discs of 2 mm thickness are inserted between stetho chest piece and skin. Number of discs needed to completely drown the sounds and make them inaudible is taken as end point. If 5 discs are needed it is D5 (the Lancet 1981) (Figs 2.44 and 2.46).

Apex Impulse

Important information about left ventricular function can be gathered by simple, but careful, palpation of the cardiac apex impulse. Stapleton and Groves discussed the various nuances of precordial palpation in an extensive review. If one excludes extracardiac causes of apex impulse displacement, such as pectus excavatum and pneumothorax, the leftward displacement of the supine apex impulse implies heart disease. It is important to observe both duration and amplitude of the apex impulse. A sustained systolic outward impulse indicates reduced myocardial contractility, while an increase in amplitude alone may be present with normal myocardial function.

Mills and Kastor have attempted to establish a quantitative grading system of cardiac palpation.

They examined 133 subjects who were placed in a 45 degree left lateral decubitus position with the left arm extended. The apex impulse was graded according to duration (D) and force (F).

Duration (requires simultaneous palpation and auscultation).

D1: The apex impulse retracts immediately after the first heart sound.
D2: The impulse retracts in the first half of systole.
D3: The impulse retracts in the latter half of systole.
D4: The impulse retracts with or after the second heart sound.

Force

F1: The faint apex impulse does not lift the lightly held finger above the chest wall.
F2: The lightly held finger is lifted, but a firmly held one is not.
F3: The firmly held finger is displaced a few millimeters.
F4: The markedly increased apex impulse makes it difficult to maintain the finger or stethoscope immobile over the cardiac apex impulse.

Conn et al studied the cardiac apex impulses in 50 patients who underwent subsequent left ventricular angiographic evaluation. The physical examination proved quite sensitive in detecting left ventricular hypertrophy than did either the electrocardiogram or the chest roentgenogram.

Paradoxical Pulses: Kussmaul coined the term 'paradoxical pulse" over a century ago in reference to the clinical situation in constrictive pericarditis in which there is an incongruity of regular heartbeat and irregular pulse. The latter, in spite of the apparent irregularity, "decreases and disappears with repetitive regularity". In modern days, the terms are used to describe a reduction in systolic blood pressure of at least 10 mm Hg during inspiration. The term is confusing since a lesser decrease of blood pressure is physiologic, whereas the term 'paradoxical' would suggest that the normal response was an increase in blood pressure during inspiration. Adding to the confusion in terminology. Massumi et al have described such an inspiratory rise in arterial systolic and diastolic pressures in certain clinical conditions, calling it 'reversed pulsus paradoxus. This entity may be observed in idiopathic hypertrophic subaortic stenosis, isorhythmic ventricular rhythms, and during intermittent positive—pressure breathing in subjects with heart failure.

The mechanism of the physiologic fall of systolic blood pressure during inspiration is related to a reduced left ventricular stroke volume during inspiration. This reduction comes from the pooling of blood in the pulmonary vasculature because of the reduced intrapleural and intrathoracic pressure (which offsets the augmented venous return and increased right ventricular volume). In pulsus paradoxus (> 10 mm Hg fall in systolic blood pressure during inspiration), right ventricular filling and left ventricular emptying are interfered with because of a nonyielding pericardial sac, accentuating the physiologic inspiratory imbalance of stroke volumes of the two ventricles. Pulsus paradoxus can also be observed in severe asthma (in which left ventricular performance is hindered by the increased intrapulmonary pressure) or in right sided heart failure, when venous return is hampered.

Reversed pulsus paradoxus (or paradoxical pulsus paradoxus, to go from the sublime to the ridiculous) may have the following mechanisms, varying according to the underlying clinical situations. In idiopathic hypertrophic subaortic stenosis (IHSS) a Valsalva-like effect may decrease left ventricular volume on expiration, hence lowering the blood pressure as compared to systolic levels. In intermittent positive pressure breathing (IPPB), the blood is squeezed out of the pulmonary capillaries and venules during positive pressure inspiration, augmenting left ventricular stroke volume and systolic blood pressure. With isorhythmic ventricular rhythm perhaps the accelerated heart rate during inspiration, permits atrial 'capture' for a few beats, increasing left ventricular volume and output during inspiration.

Systemic Manifestations

Sinus tachycardia, leukocytosis and acceleration of the sedimentation rate. These systemic signs of tissue necrosis usually appear 24-48 hours after the onset of the initial pain and are related to the amount of tissue that has undergone necrosis. They therefore serve as an estimate of the extent of infarction. The delayed systemic response is also helpful in differentiating acute myocardial infarction from such conditions as pneumonia or acute pericarditis, in which systemic abnormalities are present at the onset of illness.

Clinical Findings in Case of Acute Myocardial Infarction

A. Symptoms

1. *Pain:* Pain is the classic dominant feature of acute myocardial infarction that compels the patient in seek help. It is similar in quality to angina pectoris and may be described as heaviness or tightness or a great weight sitting on the chest. The pain is similar to ordinary angina in location and radiation, although it may radiate more widely than angina of effort and the patient recognizes that the discomfort has changed in its distribution. Not only it may radiate more widely to the lower jaw and teeth, neck, left shoulder, upper back, or down the left arm to the two fingers innervated by the ulnar nerve (which of course it may do with angina of effort), but it may also involve the upper posterior thoracic area and the patient may think there is an orthopedic problem. The pain is more severe than that of angina of effort, does not subside with rest, builds up rapidly but not instantaneously, may wax and wane, and may reach maximum severity in a few minutes. Nitroglycerin has little or no effect, which will be obvious to a patient with angina who has previously found nitroglycerin to be effective in less than 1 minute. The pain may last for hours if unrelieved by narcotics and may be unbearable. The severity of the chest pain is not related to the severity of the infarct or to its size and the physician must not be misled into considering the event a minor one because the symptoms are not devastating.

2. *Sweating, weakness, and apprehension:* The patient often breaks out into a cold sweat, feels weak and apprehensive, and moves about, seeking a position of comfort in contrast to the discomfort of angina of effort, in which the patient's instinct is to stand still or to sit or lie down.

3. *Light headedness, dyspnea, and hypotension:* In association with the pain and sweating, the patient may feel weak, faint, and lightheaded. Syncope may occur if there is a rapid onset of ventricular tachycardia or fibrillation or an atrioventricular conduction defect with a Stokes Adams attack. Syncope and manifestations of cerebral infarction are presumably the effects of decreased cardiac output on a compromised carotid or cerebral arterial supply to the brain. Ventricular arrhythmias in the first few hours after an acute infarction may cause hypotension because of the pain and fear engendered by the infarct. The myocardium often responds to acute ischemia with variable electrophysiologic changes of excitability and refractoriness, increased vulnerability to ventricular ectopia and ventricular fibrillation.

4. *Nausea, vomiting, and indigestion:* Nausea and vomiting are not rare and may be due to severe pain, vagal stimulation, so the abrupt fall in cardiac output with resulting general cellular

hypoperfusion. The discomfort may extend into the epigastrium and be associated with sensations of indigestion and bloating, so that the patient takes antacids for supposed acute indigestion, but without benefit. In retrospect, the patient may often be aware that there was similar milder discomfort in the central chest hours, days, or sometimes a week or so prior to the acute severe extent.

5. *Pulmonary edema and left ventricular failure:* In 10–20% of cases, the pain is minor and may be misinterpreted or overshadowed by the presence of acute pulmonary edema, rapidly developing left ventricular failure, profound weakness, shock, dyspnea or cough or wheezing of acute left ventricular failure.

6. *Retrospective diagnosis:* In perhaps 10% of cases, the initial symptoms are mild enough so that the diagnosis is only recognized in retrospect, when an ECG is taken months later and evidence or previous acute infarction is discovered that was not previously present. This is particularly true in patients with autonomic nervous system dysfunction due to diabetes mellitus. The patient may fail to realize that myocardial infarction has occurred because the pain lasts only 30 minutes and is unrelated to effort, with onset at rest or even during sleep. A patient with previous angina of effort will recognize the unusual features, particularly the severity, radiation, and duration of the discomfort and its failure to respond to nitroglycerin, however, a patient who has not had angina of effort may interpret the discomfort as indigestion or musculoskeletal disease or may merely complain of feeling unwell.

B. Signs: The signs of acute myocardial infarction may be trivial, or the patient may be at the point of death when first seen. The clinical picture is related to the size and extent of the infarction, the presence of previous infarction with left ventricular dysfunction and the adequacy of the collateral circulation.

1. *Initial signs:* The initial signs may be more severe than those found 1–2 hours later, especially if the patient has had a ventricular arrhythmia, marked bradycardia with poor output, or abrupt left ventricular failure, which subsided as compensatory reflex mechanisms, came into play.

2. *Signs in mild cases:* In mild cases the patient may appear well. The skin may be dry and the pulse and blood pressure normal and there may be no signs of failure, the patient complaining only of prolonged substernal discomfort.

3. *Signs in more severe cases:* In more severe cases, the patient appears acutely ill, may have marked hypotension with low cardiac output, tachycardia, cold clammy, sweaty skin, and a gray (ashen) appearance due to peripheral cyanosis. If cerebral perfusion is impaired, the patient may be mentally dull and confused and may have either tachycardia or bradycardia depending upon whether the baroreceptor response to low cardiac output predominates or impairment of perfusion to the sinus node or vagal reflexes produces sinus bradycardia. At the onset of acute myocardial infarction, the temperature is usually normal. Fever is delayed for 24–72 hours and is due to myocardial necrosis, which takes time to develop.

A Combination of shock and cardiac failure: A patient with clinically apparent shock with a systolic pressure less than 80 mm Hg and a urine output less than 20 mL/h may show signs of left ventricular failure with a diastolic gallop rhythm, pulsus alternans, and bilateral rales. The gallop and rales may rapidly progress to acute pulmonary edema or right-sided congestive heart failure or may remain the same. The chest X-ray confirms left ventricular failure by haziness in the central lung fields if there is transudation into the alveoli or redistribution of flow to the upper lobe if there is interstitial edema, Kerley's B lines may also occur after some days but may be out of phase with the clinical signs and there may be hemodynamic evidence of raised pulmonary artery diastolic pressure. At any time, there may be a discrepancy between the radiologic evidence of left ventricular failure and the pulmonary artery diastolic pressure. Although the radiologic signs lag behind the hemodynamic ones, X-ray offers valuable evidence of cardiac failure. When the pulmonary artery wedge pressure is normal, the great majority of patients have no radiographic evidence of left ventricular failure or pulmonary congestion. When patients have a high degree of raised wedge pressure (more than 25 mm Hg radiologic changes of pulmonary congestion are almost always present (Kostuk, 1973).

The venous pressure may be raised, but this may be difficult to recognize because of the venous constriction resulting from the intense sympathetic discharge caused by the low cardiac output; yet when hemodynamic studies are done, the right atrial pressure is elevated. If the signs of shock are delayed, venous construction out of proportion to arteriolar construction may lead to transudation of fluid out of the capillaries, and the patient may be hypovolemic in which instance the right atrial pressure is low and volume repletion is indicated.

Clinical Findings of Angina

The term angina denotes a specific type of chest discomfort associated with myocardial ischemia and is now used only in that sense. Pain in the chest is one of the most common complaints the physician is called upon to assess, and it is important for the physician to be able to differentiate the various causes of chest pain because of the potential seriousness of the symptom, with its connotation of disability and death.

A. Induction of Angina by Procedure: That increases the metabolic demands of the heart.

1. *Interpretation of pain:* The interpretation of the symptom must be based on the history alone, because about one-fourth of patients have no objective clinical findings of coronary atherosclerosis to support the history. The diagnosis may be simple or extremely difficult. The diagnosis of angina is more probable if there is ECG evidence of myocardial ischemia, a history of myocardial infarction, or other data establishing the presence of ischemia such as ECG changes induced by exercise, areas of hypoperfusion seen on radioisotopic scans, or abnormalities of left ventricular wall motion seen on echocardiogram. Even the known concurrence of established coronary disease does not rule out other causes of chest pain. However, the likelihood that an uncertain history represents angina is increased by resting or induced myocardial ischemia, the presence of other atherosclerotic manifestations such as intermittent claudication, cerebral ischemic attacks or bruits over the major arteries. Similarly, a strong family history of early coronary disease or a personal history of hypertension, diabetes, or hypercholesterolemia increases the likelihood of coronary disease in a patient with equivocal chest discomfort. Dyspnea, fatigue, cardiac enlargement, and cardiac failure are not sufficient to establish a diagnosis of angina because they may be due to many other causes.

2. *Pain as support for the diagnosis of angina:* If the patient's chest discomfort is in fact induced by procedures (such as exercise, rapid atrial pacing, or isoproterenol infusion) that increase myocardial oxygen demand and if production of chest discomfort is associated with ECG evidence of

myocardial ischemia, a transiently raised left ventricular, end-diastolic pressure with evidence of left ventricular dysfunction, or isotopic demonstration of hypoperfusion in an area of the myocardium, the diagnosis is strongly supported in doubtful cases, 12 to 24 hours continuous ECG tape recordings (Holter) can be used to look for the presence of ischemic ST segments during episodes of pain. Significant ischemic ST segments may be found in patients who have angina pectoris even in the absence of pain.

a. Coronary arteriography is rarely justified for diagnosis alone except in unusual circumstances.

3. *Characteristics of angina:* The characteristics of angina pain have been well described in the past by Herberden (1768), Herrick (1912), and Levine (1929). The discomfort is described by most patients as a sensation of tightness or pressure starting in the center of the chest and radiating to the lower jaw and to the inner surface of the left arm and to the outer two fingers.

a. *Precipitating factors:* The pain is induced by anything that increases the oxygen requirements of the myocardium; examples are exercise, sexual activity, emotional stress, cold weather, wind, a large meal, anemia, an increase in blood pressure, tachycardia, high altitude, or decreased oxygen content of the inspired air. The essential features of the history include the circumstances that precipitate or relieve the discomfort and the characteristics of the discomfort itself, including its location, radiation, and duration. The essential feature is that the discomfort is precipitated in circumstances that increase the oxygen demands of the myocardium, the most common circumstances occurs during walking, especially when hurrying or walking up an incline or a flight of stairs.

b. Prinzmetal (1959) described one type of angina occurring at rest as 'variant angina' it is thought to be due to coronary vasoconstriction. Variant angina occasionally occurs in patients with minimal coronary stenosis or spasms, but most cases have substantial coronary artery lesions.

1. Usually, however, the discomfort of angina occurs during exertion and subsides promptly if the patient stands or sits quietly. If other factors upset the balance between myocardial oxygen supply and demand, less activity is required to produce angina, especially after meals, during times of emotional excitement or on exposure to a cold wind. Heavy meals and strong emotion can provide an attack even with trivial exertion.

a. The discomfort of angina of effort lasts but a short time if the effort is discontinued usually less than 10–15 minutes and usually much less. The discomfort develops and subsides fairly quickly but not abruptly. If the effort is continued unabated, the discomfort increases until the patient must stop. Occasionally, a patient learns to decrease activity until discomfort subsides and thus 'walks through' the angina.

B. **Quality of Angina Pain:** Patients describe angina pain as pressing, squeezing, a tightness, a weight on the chest rarely, as though the chest is in a vise. They may describe it as burning and may have difficulty finding the right word but will convey the type of discomfort by pressing on the chest with both hands, as first noted by Levine (1958). Many patients use the term discomfort or distress rather than pain and will answer 'No' to the question, 'Do you have or have you had chest pain?' The pain is rarely stabbing, lancinating, pointed, or piercing.

C. **Location of Angina Pain:** The pain usually covers a fairly broad area in the central chest and has diffuse, ill-defined edges. Although it may be dominantly left precordial, it usually involves the central chest and is rarely solely left precordial, lateral, or epigastric. Patients may think that the pain is in the abdomen, but, when asked to define the site on the nude chest and abdomen, will point to the lower mid chest. Nonanginal 'abdominal' pain is below the xiphoid and involves only the epigastrium and not the chest. Anginal pain may involve the lower area of the sternum and extend into the epigastrium. Rarely, there is localized tenderness during or between attacks in contrast to patients with musculoskeletal or radicular disease, in whom this is common.

D. **Radiation of Angina Pain:** The pain radiates to the lower jaw (never to the upper jaw), upper neck, left shoulder, and inner surface of the arm to the ulnar surface of the hand in the fourth and fifth fingers. It may be felt only as a sensation of pressure across the volar surface of the wrist. Rarely, a patient with angina may go to the dentist with a 'toothache' or to an orthopedician complaining of upper back pain. Chest discomfort is often the only symptom, but there may be associated dyspnea if there is some element of left ventricular failure during episodes of pain.

The pain or discomfort of angina pectoris is a visceral pain from the heart referred from C_8-T_1 segmental dermatomes. Small pain fibers run with the autonomic nerves and enter the spinal cord in the C_8 and T_1 segments. As with all visceral pain, if it is poorly localized. The diaphragm is innervated by C4 and neck pain may be related to the cutaneous pattern of this segment. The thumb is innervated by C5 and C6 and is rarely involved in angina pain.

E. **Ease of production of pain:** The ease of production of the pain during efforts varies on different days, often depending upon how the patient feels emotionally, whether the patient is out of doors or not, how cold and windy it is, and how much time has elapsed since eating. All of these factors increase the work of the heart. When patients with 'stable' or chronic angina are exercised in a comfortable laboratory on an empty stomach in a relaxed state of mind, the amount of exercise required to induce pain is fairly constant (within 10%).

F. **Patient Response to Pain:** Patients learn to avoid pain by recognizing the earliest manifestations of pressure or tightness in the chest when they are walking or start to get excited. Most patients must slow down or stop walking and stand still, since otherwise the pain worsens until they are forced to stop. A patient may have discomfort hurrying to the bus in the morning but may find that a similar amount of effort later in the morning or in the afternoon causes no discomfort. Similarly, an individual may have discomfort during the first one or two holes of golf and then play the rest of the game in comfort. This uncommon second wind phenomenon is presumably explicable as local vasodilatation caused by metabolites accumulated during the ischemic pain period.

G. **Coronary Spasm (Prinzmetal's Variant Angina):** Coronary artery spasm, suggested in the past as a possible cause of variant angina pectoris, has in recent years been found to contribute to a greater extent than previously believed to a variety of manifestations of ischemic cardiac disease (Hillis, 1978). Variant angina, described by Prinzmetal in 1959, was attributed to spasm of the large coronary arteries because coronary arteriograms were frequently negative and because there was elevation and not depression of the ST segment in the ECG during the pain.

a. Prinzmetal's variant angina differs from ordinary angina of effort in that it is more apt to occur at rest than with effort, may occur at odd times during the day or night (even awakening patients from sleep) and is more likely to be associated with various types of arrhythmias or conduction defects. The ST segment is more commonly elevated rather than depressed, as occurs during angina of effort. There are hemodynamic differences as well. Both variant angina and angina of effort respond rapidly to sublingual nitrates. Patients with variant angina usually have no history of previous myocardial infarction, whereas those with the usual angina of effort have such a history in approximately half of cases. Variant angina is more common in women under age 50, whereas angina of effort is uncommon in women of this age in the absence of severe hypercholesterolemia, hypertension, or diabetes mellitus.

b. Signs: Examination is often completely negative in patients with angina pectoris who have not had a previous myocardial infarction and who show no evidence of hypertensive or aortic valve disease. The heart may be normal in size, the left ventricular cardiac impulse may be normal, and there may be no abnormal third or fourth sounds. However, there may be associated evidence of atherosclerosis such as decreased pulsations or bruits over the major arteries. The ocular fundi are usually normal unless the patient has hypertension or diabetes. During an attack, the systolic and diastolic blood pressures are usually significantly elevated, and there may be a third heart sound, pulsus alternans, or transient pulmonary rales.

Differential Diagnosis

The differential diagnosis of chest pain requires great skill in history taking. The physician can usually decide that the pain is or is not angina, but in some cases even the most careful and thoughtful inquiry may leave the issue in doubt. Chest pain in someone with coronary disease is not necessarily angina.

A. **Psychophysiologic Reactions:** Psychophysiologic cardiovascular reactions are a loosely defined group of disorders having in common dull aching chest pains often described as 'heart pain', lasting hours or days, often aggravated by exertion but not promptly relieve by rest. Darting, knifelike pains of momentary duration at the apex or over the precordium are often present also. Emotional tension and fatigue make the pain worse. Dyspnea of the hyperventilation variety, palpitations, fatigue, and headache are also usually present. Constant exhaustion is a frequent complaint.

B. **Anterior Chest Wall Syndrome:** This disorder is characterized by sharply localized tenderness of intercostal muscles, and pressure at these sites reproduces the chest pain. Sprain or inflammation of the chondrocostal junctions, which may be warm, swollen, and red (so-called Tietze's syndrome), may result in diffuse chest pain which is also reproduced by the local pressure. Intercostal neuritis (herpes zoster, diabetes mellitus) may confuse the diagnosis.

Xiphoid tenderness and lower sternal pain may arise from and be reproduced by pressure on the xiphoid process.

Any of the above may also occur in a patient with angina.

C. **Degenerative Thoracic or Cervical Spine Disease:** Cervical or thoracic spine disease (degenerative disk disease, postural strain, 'arthritis) involving the dorsal roots produces sudden sharp, severe chest pain similar to angina in location and radiation but related to specific movements of the neck or spine, recumbency, straining, or lifting, and there are usually sensory changes in the skin. Pain due to cervical thoracic disk disease involves the outer or dorsal aspect of the arm, thumb, and index fingers there than the ring and little fingers, as in angina pectoris.

D. Gastrointestinal Disorders: Peptic ulcer, chronic chotecystitis, cardiospasm, and functional gastrointestinal disease are often suspected because some patients indisputably obtain relief from angina by blocking. In these disorders, symptoms are related to food intake rather than physical exertion. X-ray and fluoroscopic study are helpful in diagnosis. The pain is relieved by appropriate diet and drug therapy.

Hiatal hernia is characterized by lower chest and upper abdominal pain after heavy meals occurring in recumbency, upon bending over, or made worse with the acid or alcohol test. The pain is relieved by bland diet, antacids, the semi-Fowler position, and walking.

E. Shoulder Origin of Pain: Degenerative and inflammatory lesions of the left shoulder or cervical rib and the scalenus anticus syndrome differ from angina in that the pain is precipitated by movement of the arm and shoulder, paresthesias are present in the left arm and postural exercises and pillow support to the shoulders in bed gives relief.

F. Pain of Pulmonary Hypertension: Tight mitral stenosis or pulmonary hypertension resulting from chronic pulmonary disease can on occasion produce chest pain which is indistinguishable from that of angina pectoris, including ST segment depression. The clinical findings of mitral stenosis or of lung disease are evident, and the ECG invariably discloses right axis deviation or right ventricular hypertrophy. Pulmonary embolism must also be considered.

G. Spontaneous Pneumothorax: Spontaneous pneumothorax may cause chest pain as well as dyspnea and create confusion with angina pectoris as well as myocardial infarction.

H. Pericarditis.

Clinical Features of Hypertension

The clinical, laboratory, and radiologic findings relate to (1) the height of the blood pressure; (2) the involvement of 'target organs' such as the heart, brain, kidneys, eyes, and peripheral arteries; (3) the presence of vascular complications such as cardiac failure, myocardial infarction, cerebral infarction, cerebral hemorrhage, atherosclerosis elsewhere, and dissection of the aorta; and (4) evidence of secondary 'curable' hypertension.

A. Symptoms: Primary hypertension early in its course is usually an asymptomatic disorder compatible with well-being for many years. Vague symptoms of nonspecific headache, dizziness, fatigue, and pounding of the heart may be present in hypertensive patients (often only after patients learn that they have the condition) but are no more frequent than in some groups of patients with normotension. The frequency of vague symptoms that resemble those seen in psychoneurotic disorders has led investigators such as Ayman (1940) to conclude that these nonspecific symptoms in patients with mild hypertension are functional in origin and not organic. Screening of adult population groups often reveals the blood pressure to be elevated in vigorous subjects who have no symptoms whatever.

1. *Headaches:* When hypertension is more severe, especially if it is the accelerated variety (with rapid rise in pressure and hemorrhages or exudates in the fundi, considered premalignant) throbbing suboccipital headaches, worse in the morning and subsiding during the day, are common. In malignant hypertension in association with visual disturbances, the headaches can be severe and most difficult to relieve except by reduction

of the blood pressure. In contrast with the typical hypertensive headache, the usual tension headache is more apt to be frontal and nonthrobbing; the differentiation is often difficult.

2. *Heart failure:* When left ventricular dilatation and early left ventricular failure occur in patients with compensatory cardiac hypertrophy, symptoms include progressively more severe dyspnea on exertion, paroxysmal nocturnal dyspnea, and orthopnea. If coronary heart disease is also present, as it commonly is, patients may complain of angina pectoris or may develop myocardial infarction. Left ventricular failure resulting from the combination of increased work of the left ventricle due to hypertension and associated coronary heart disease is frequent and makes precise distinction between causative factors difficult. Cardiac failure from modest elevations of blood pressure alone does not usually occur. When the raised blood pressure is greater, and particularly when it occurs abruptly, as in malignant hypertension, cardiac failure may occur in the absence of coronary heart disease and is rapidly reversed when the blood pressure is lowered. Hypertensive patients with cardiac hypertrophy often develop symptoms and signs of cardiac failure if the sodium intake is abruptly increased, as with ingestion of baking soda. Alka-Seltzer, or a high sodium diet; these patients often respond rapidly to treatment. Cardiac failure is an uncommon cause of death in the well-managed patient unless it follows the complications of myocardial infarction. Typical electrocardiographic examples of left ventricular hypertrophy and its reversal are illustrated.

3. *Renal symptoms*: Although nephrosclerosis is a common findings on pathologic examination (by either necropsy or renal biopsy), renal failure is not common unless hypertension is accelerated, or malignant. Patients with severe hypertension may develop nocturia or more rarely, intermittent hematuria. In nonaccelerated cases, renal blood flow and glomerular filtration rate may be somewhat decreased, but renal failure and azotemia are rare. If accelerated, or malignant, hypertension occurs, however, necrotic lesions in the arterioles and narrowed interlobular arteries may significantly decrease the renal blood flow and glomerular filtration rate; renal function may deteriorate rapidly over a period of weeks or months.

The most common cause of death in malignant hypertension is renal failure, determination of renal function is essential in all patients with hypertension because, as will be discussed in the section on prognosis, it is important to lower the blood pressure before renal failure has occurred.

4. *Central nervous system symptoms:* Older patients with hypertension and associated cerebral and carotid artery sclerosis may develop any of the clinical manifestations of atherosclerosis of the arteries and arterioles to the head that might be excepted from the pathologic findings described above. Patients may develop severe headache, confusion, coma, convulsions, blurred vision, transient neurologic signs, ataxia, or neurologic deficit due to cerebral infarction or hemorrhage. If the blood pressure rises abruptly, patients may develop acute cerebral symptoms such as somnolence, coma, confusion, or convulsions, collectively known as hypertensive encephalopathy presumably due to cerebral spasm and cerebral edema and these may be quickly reversed with rapidly acting antihypertensive agents. More

commonly, however, when these severe cerebral symptoms develop, a vascular accident has occurred rather than cerebral spasm and edema.

Acute interruption of the blood supply to a localized area of the brain causes a focal neurologic deficit (stroke). The most common type is thrombotic cerebral infarction; the least common is cerebral embolism; and intermediate in frequency is cerebral hemorrhage from rupture of a berry aneurysm or a Charcot Bouchard microaneurysm of one of the small arteries of the brain. Impaired blood supply may be either intra or extracranial and may occur at a wide variety of sites in any of the extracranial arteries, especially the internal carotid, the basilar, and the vestibular arteries. The intracranial sites for atherosclerosis are dominantly the middle cerebral artery and the circle of Willis.

5. *Claudication:* When atherosclerosis involves the aorta and the arteries of the lower extremities, patients may present with intermittent claudication, and hypertension is only noted incidentally.

6. *Chest pain:* Severe chest pain radiating to the back, followed by interruption of the arterial supply to the head, neck, back, and lower extremities, occurs after dissection of the aorta, in type I (see later under discussion of dissection) involving the ascending aorta, aortic insufficiency may result. Hypertension may be noted only incidentally in patients who present with severe chest pain simulating acute myocardial infarction or acute aortic insufficiency.

As indicated under heart failure above, coronary heart disease frequently complicates hypertension. Patients may develop angina pectoris or myocardial infarction, chest pain may not be due to dissection of the aorta but to angina pectoris and myocardial ischemia.

B. Signs: The physical signs in hypertension are related to the underlying causes of the hypertension, its duration and severity, the blood pressure itself, the presence and degree of involvement of the target organs, and complications resulting from vascular involvement.

1. *Blood pressure (Figs 2.26 and 2.47)*
   i. *Cuff width:* The blood pressure should be taken with a mercury manometer or a well-calibrated aneroid manometer in both arms and in the legs, using a cuff at least 12 cm wide in most persons. A wide leg cuff (14–15 cm) must be used on the arm if the patient is obese or very muscular, with a large upper arm circumference. The cuff should be at least two-thirds as wide as the upper arm is long. Errors are frequently made in diagnosing hypertension if the cuff is too narrow and does not adequately compress the brachial artery. The basic principle is that a cuff which is too narrow for the size of the arm gives readings that are falsely high.

   ii. *Measuring blood pressure:* The patient should be relaxed, warm, and unhurried, and the physicians's routine should include allowing the patient to adjust to the examining room. The pressure must be taken in both arms to avoid discrepancies caused by atherosclerosis of the subclavian artery; the arm in which the pressure is to be taken on subsequent occasions should be noted.

   Accurate technic in taking the blood pressure is essential, and nurses, field workers, and others must be carefully instructed in placement of the rubber bag over the artery and the speed of inflation and deflation is measuring the pressure.

iii. *Home measurement and ambulatory blood pressure recordings:* The patient or a member of the patient's family can be taught to take blood pressure readings at home. Systolic and diastolic pressures taken 3 or 4 times a day can be averaged into weekly mean pressures. Mean blood pressures so obtained have been shown to be reliable by Page, Dustan and their associates at the Cleveland Clinic (Barvo, 1975) not only in establishing the presence of hypertension but also in providing a baseline to evaluate treatment. Ambulatory blood pressure readings can be taken with portable self-recording equipment in order to eliminate the pressor effect of the physician and the medical environment. Mean ambulatory pressures lower than mean office pressures occurred in 85% of 675 untreated hypertensive patients. Mean ambulatory pressures averaged 13% lower than office pressures for the total population, with a wide scatter, even though the correlation coefficient of the 2 methods of measuring pressures is 0.67. These ancillary techniques are usually needed only when raised pressures are mild to moderate (~ 180/105 mm Hg) and are not necessary when the pressures are considerably raised on 2 or 3 occasions but normal on others.

Examples of the use of ambulatory blood pressure monitoring.

a. Even when office blood pressures are more than moderately raised, an occasional patient will have essentially normal readings at home when pressures are taken by someone other than a physician or when pressures are recorded by a portable apparatus. Prolonged recording with intra-arterial or automatic devices especially during sleep, is valuable in assessing hypertension and may demonstrate a marked decrease in pressures in the early morning hours.

b. Considerable care must be taken to establish the diagnosis of hypertension before instituting treatment because treatment is usually a lifelong process. Treatment is rarely urgent in the absence of severe or accelerated hypertension.

c. Variations in measurement: The body position of the patient is also important; when the patient sits or stands, the diastolic pressure may increase over recumbent levels because of stimulation of the carotid and aortic baroreceptors. The systolic pressure may stay the same or occasionally may fall slightly in the standing position, but it may increase in the sitting position. If the patient is hypovolemic, as a result of administration of diuretics or has postural hypotension from antihypertensive agents interfering with adrenergic transmission, the systolic and diastolic pressure may be considerably lower in the sitting and standing position than in recumbency. In autonomic insufficiency, postural hypotension is accompanied by little or no tachycardia in contrast to the marked tachycardia that occurs in postural hypotension due to hypovolemia. Because of the transient rise in pressure that occurs with the stress of the examination in the sometimes threatening environment of the doctor's office, a raised pressure must be present on at least three different occasions of measurement before one considers the pressure to be representative. Sometimes the pressure is so variable that it is elevated on one occasion but well thin the normal range on another; this may occur in 10–20%

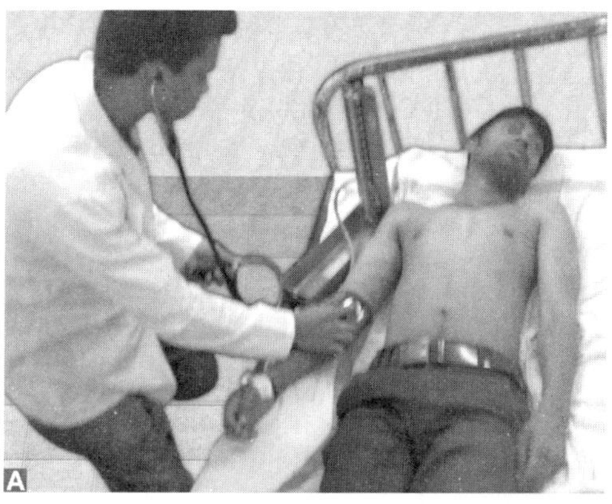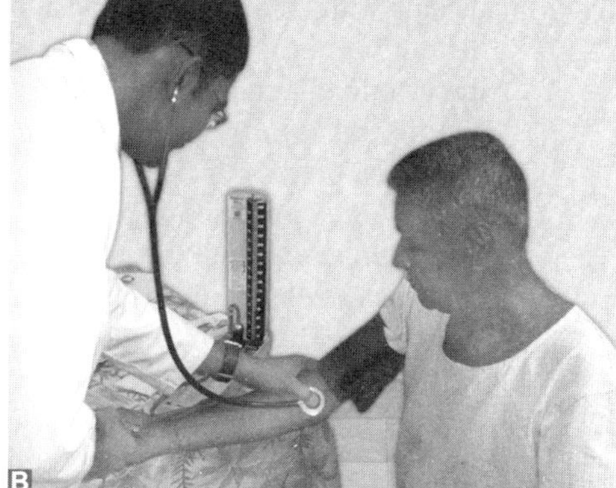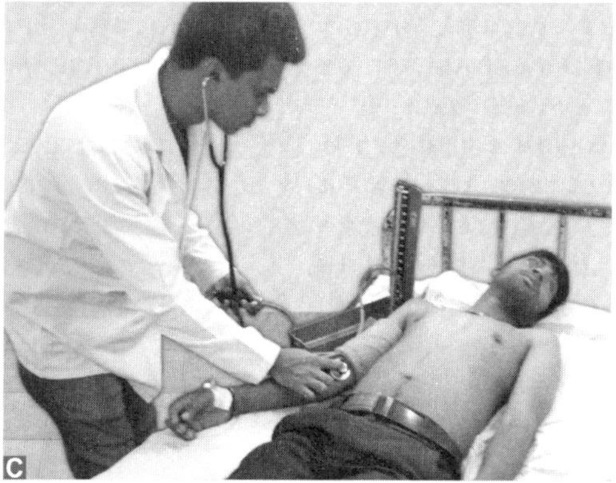

Figs 2.47A to C: Blood pressure—Measurement

of individuals during any short period of time. It then becomes necessary to obtain frequent office, home, or ambulatory blood pressure readings over a period of weeks or even months or to have readings taken by a nurse in the office under relaxed circumstances without the doctor being present.

2. *Signs in target organs:* Particular emphasis should be placed on the following signs related to an assessment of the presence and degree of involvement of the target organs affected by hypertension or by the presence or absence of vascular complications of hypertension.

   i. *Retinas:* In examining the retinas one should note particularly the degree of narrowing or irregularity of the arterioles, the presence of arteriovenous defects ('nicking' or 'nipping'), the presence of flame shaped or circular hemorrhages, fluffy cotton wool exudates, or the presence of papilledema with blurring of the temporal edge or elevation of the optic disk. Keith, Wagener, and Barker (1939) have classified the retinal changes as follows (called Keith-Wagener (KW) changes).

   KW 1: Minimal arteriolar narrowing, irregularity of the lumen, and increased light reflex.

   KW II: More marked narrowing with focal spasm, more marked irregularity, and arteriovenous nicking with changes in course and distention of the vein as it crosses the arteriole. The arteriole and the venule travel in the same sheath, and when there is thickening of the arteriole it compresses the venule.

KW III: In addition to the arteriolar changes noted previously, multiple flame shaped hemorrhages and fluffy 'cotton wool' exudates are scattered throughout the retinas. These are due to localized axon swellings and swollen nerve fibers in avascular areas. Hard, very small, sharply defined, translucent exudates are due to exudation in a different part of the retina, are of lesser significance, and do not indicate acute arteriolar damage.

KW IV: Any of the above with the addition of papilledema with blurring of the temporal side of the optic disk and elevation of the disk. Caution should be exercised in interpreting blurring of the nasal edge of the disk as being due to papilledema. Old, healed papilledema in the absence of current elevation of the disk margins is often revealed by the presence of small collateral vessels crossing the edge of the disk.

Benign hypertension is the rule when KW I and KW II are present, whereas KW III and KW IV are associated with accelerated, or malignant, hypertension. When malignant hypertension develops abruptly with only a short history of hypertension, patients may have hemorrhages, exudates, or papilledema in the absence of arteriolar changes or arteriovenous nicking.

The Keith-Wagener classification has some deficiencies, particularly in the differentiation of hypertensive from atherosclerotic changes in KW II and in the interpretation of single hemorrhages and 'hard' exudates. The two processes, hypertension and atherosclerosis, are independent entities, but hypertension accelerates atherosclerosis. When the arterioles are very narrowed and irregular and compress the venules, the findings are a combination of the two pathologic processes and are not due to hypertension alone; therefore, arteriovenous nicking indicates the presence of atherosclerosis and, by inference, a longer duration of the hypertensive process. The fundal changes of accelerated hypertension are an urgent indication for immediate and vigorous antihypertensive therapy.

ii. Heart: Examination of the heart and blood vessels may reveal evidence of left ventricular hypertrophy, left ventricular failure, or involvement of the various arteries by atherosclerosis. As shown by Traube in the late 19th century, the best sign of left ventricular hypertrophy is a left ventricular heave a localized sustained lift of the left ventricular impulse. Because concentric hypertrophy is the rule prior to dilatation and left ventricular failure, the heart is not displaced onto the left unless cardiac failure is present. The decreased distensibility of the thick left ventricle commonly procedures a presystolic gallop (S4); this does not indicate cardiac failure but is a sign of decreased left ventricular compliance. The presence of a left ventricular heave and an S4 indicates established left ventricular hypertrophy and usually long-standing disease.

iii. Blood vessels: The jugular venous pulse is usually normal in the absence of right ventricular failure, the carotid pulses are usually normal in volume and upstroke unless the patient has coarctation of the aorta, in which case the carotid pulse is unusually prominent and jerky. The presence of bruits over the carotid should always be sought as a possible clue to the presence of atherosclerotic disease of the internal carotid arteries. The presence or absence of pulmonary rales is valuable in recognizing early left ventricular failure. If the failure is more obvious and more severe, pulsus alternans may be noted. Particular note should be made of the volume and character of all the pulses and their symmetry on the two sides. This serves not only to demonstrate coarctation of the aorta if the pulses of the lower extremities are weak and delayed as compared to those of the radials but also to provide a baseline in the event the patient develops chest pain, with variation in the various pulses suggesting aortic dissection. The presence or absence of bruits should be sought, especially over the femoral and popliteal arteries, to determine the presence of atherosclerosis of these vessels. Bruits should be sought in the epigastrium and in the flanks, since they may provide dues that suggest renovascular hypertension. Examination of the abdominal aorta may reveal an aneurysm as a complication of concomitant atherosclerosis. Careful palpation below each rib should be done in a search for pulsating intercostal arteries, which are prominent in coarctation of the aorta and serve as collateral vessels to arteries below the coarctated site.

iv. Central nervous system signs: Examination for evidence of residual neurologic deficit from previous cerebral infarction may be fruitful. There may be a positive Babinski or Hoffman reflex, hemiparesis, hemiplegia, or hemianopsia. The presence of ataxia may indicate involvement of the posterior-inferior cerebellar artery.

v. Endocrine dysfunction: The patient should be examined for signs suggesting any of several types of endocrine abnormalities, Cushing's syndrome is suspected if there is central trunk obesity, hirsutism, acne purple striae, moon facies, and thin skin with ecchymoses. Primary aldosteronism is suggested by muscular weakness, hypoactive deep tendon reflexes, and diminished or absent vasomotor circulatory reflexes. Pheochromocytoma is suspected if an attack of headache, sweating, palpitations, and a markedly increased blood pressure is induced by an examination over the upper abdomen that presses on a tumor.

v. **Coarctation of the aorta:** Coarctation is strongly suggested by the presence of weak or delayed femoral pulses in comparison with the radial pulses, the presence of a basal systolic ejection murmur transmitted to the interscapular area, and palpable collateral intercostals arteries along the inferior rib margins and scapular borders.

vi. **Polycystic kidneys:** Polycystic kidneys are suspected if the kidneys are large and easily palpable, especially in the presence of long standing hypertension, when the kidneys would be expected to be small.

C. **Laboratory Findings:** Laboratory investigations are designed to determine the involvement of any of the target organs affected by hypertension and to recognize the presence of any evidence of secondary hypertension. (The diagnosis and details of secondary hypertension will be described later.)

Malignant Hypertension

Malignant hypertension is a syndrome characterized by a rapidly rising blood pressure (diastolic pressures usually in excess of 130 mm Hg) from any cause. Unless effective antihypertensive therapy is given promptly, there may be severe visual loss associated with hemorrhage, exudates, and papilledema of the ocular fundi; and death due to uremia, heart failure, or cerebral hemorrhage usually occurs in less than 1 year. Pathologic changes are seen in the arterioles and in the small interlobular arteries. The kidney is progressively destroyed by ischemic atrophy of the nephrons, with decrease in glomerular filtration rate and renal blood flow because of fibrinoid necrosis of the arterioles and cellular intimal proliferation of the interlobular arteries. Some patients with pathologically proved fibrinoid necrosis do not have papilledema, but they usually have hemorrhage or exudates in the fundi. Prognostic studies have shown that the 3 to 5 years mortality rate is essentially indistinguishable in untreated patients with KW III fundi as compared to those with KW IV fundi; both represent accelerated hypertension.

The rapid rise in blood pressure may cause cardiac failure within 1–2 weeks and renal failure within a month. Examination of the retinas for evidence of accelerated hypertension is necessary in all hypertensive patients, because the early stages of the malignant phase may be essentially asymptomatic, although severe headache, acute visual disturbances and gross hematuria are the usual presenting manifestations. Cardiac and renal failure may occur with great rapidity and treatment to lower the blood pressure is urgent. Patients seen early with evidence of accelerated, or malignant, hypertension may have normal renal function and even absence of proteinuria. This rapidly progresses, however, to malignant hypertension with proteinuria and azotemia and then finally to renal failure. For this reason, treatment is essential before the development of renal failure.

Malignant hypertension is a quantitatively more severe form of hypertension, and prevention is far more effective than treatment of the established or advanced disease. Accelerated, or malignant hypertension is rare in properly treated hypertensives.

The importance of prevention of the malignant phase can be outlined as follows:

Malignant hypertension is rare in the properly managed patient with benign hypertension.

Adequate follow-up and education of patient regarding compliance with therapy is essential. Stopping therapy in severe hypertension is hazardous.

Early symptoms of accelerated disease (sudden onset of visual disturbances, severe headache, gross hematuria) should trigger therapeutic treatment.

Prognosis of malignant hypertension is related to the degree of renal impairment existing when treatment began.

Treatment of severe hypertension prevents the malignant phase, early treatment of the malignant phase prevents azotemia, treatment of azotemia without uremia prevents uremia.

Mortality rate in the treatment of severe hypertension is related to the effectiveness with which the blood pressure was lowered.

Complications

Dissection of the Aorta

One of the complications of hypertension that often is unrecognized, especially in pregnant women, is dissection of the aorta. Hypertension is the presumed cause in one-third of cases of proximal and two-thirds of cases of distal dissection (Stater, 1976). Cystic medial necrosis and arteriosclerosis are much less common causes. The onset is usually acute (90% of cases), with severe instantaneous chest pain radiating to the back or abdomen combine with evidence of obstruction of the branches of the aorta and diminished or absent pulses from the carotids to the femoral arteries. The diagnosis can be established by supravalvular angiography, although it can be strongly suspected clinically and radiologically. If one records a widened aorta or a double echo in the aorta in the presence of clinical evidence of aortic root dissection, the diagnosis can also be suspected on the basis of echocardiography. The abrupt development of chest pain, aortic insufficiency, diminished or absent pulses, or the appearance of signs of 'sympathectomy' on one side and of neurologic deficit with cerebral symptoms should make one think of dissection of the aorta. The pain may be differentiated from that of acute myocardial infarction by its instantaneous onset, its severity, the absence of central pulses, and the presence of hypertension despite pain or even shock. Aortic dissection has been classified as type I, which involves the proximal ascending aorta and aortic arch, at times extending distally to the iliac arteries, type II, which involves only the ascending aorta and is sometimes combined with type I and called proximal dissection, and type III, which involves only the distal aorta beyond the left subclavian artery. Types I and II may involves the aortic valve, causing aortic insufficiency and heart failure, and are more serious than type III.

Dissection involving the distal aorta may be treated medically with intensive antihypertensive therapy (sodium nitroprusside infusion combined with propranolol and perhaps methyldopa) and surgical treatment is reserved for the patient who fails to respond. When intensive intravenous hypotensive therapy is used, the renal output must be carefully monitored and not allowed to decrease below 20 or 30 mL/h. In type I and II dissection, the mortality rate is high, aortic insufficiency may occur, and the aorta may rupture into the pericardium or pleura; after immediate lowering of the blood pressure with parenteral antihypertensive agents and establishment of the diagnosis by supravalvular aortography, surgical treatment is recommended. Without treatment, the mortality rate is very high, but with modern surgical treatment survival may be as high as 75%. Some authorities believe that nearly all patients with proximal aortic dissection should undergo operation immediately after their general condition has stabilized whereas those patients with distal dissection, because of its lesser hazard, can be monitored in the intensive care unit.

RENAL ARTERY STENOSIS

Renal artery stenosis is probably the most common cause of curable secondary hypertension, but clinical enthusiasm for seeking out the diagnosis and treating by operation has varied in recent years (Withelmsen, 1977, Tucker, 1977). This is partly because of the rarity of the condition but also because the vascular complications can often be managed by medical antihypertensive therapy in less severe cases and partly because the operation is associated with significant morbidity and mortality rates in older people with atherosclerotic renal artery stenosis due to clinical atherosclerosis elsewhere in the vascular system. Furthermore, surgical relief of the obstruction does not always cure the hypertension even in patients whose renal artery stenosis has been proved by selective renal angiography and differential renal vein renin concentration. Significant improvement occurs in about 75% of patients with fibromuscular hyperplasia and about 50% of patients with atherosclerotic renal artery stenosis.

Angioplasty of renal artery cures many cases.

CARDIAC FAILURE

Almost all cardiac diseases ultimately culminate into 'failure' left ventricular, right ventricular or both hence a clinician should be an expert in clinical recognition of cardiac failure.

Definition

Cardiac failure can be broadly defined as a state in which the heart fails to meet the varying oxygen and metabolic needs of the body under differing circumstances, or a state in which cardiac output (the ability of the heart to pump blood) is reduced relative to the metabolic demands of the body, assuming the existence of adequate venous return. The definition is arbitrary and controversial, because the phenomena of heart failure are complex and incompletely understood. If one uses a symptom such as dyspnea on exertion appearing for the first time as the manifestation signaling the onset of cardiac failure in the left ventricular disease. This criterion may be deceptive because physiologically active patients will demonstrate dyspnea earlier than patients who are sedentary and because a sedentary person with no heart disease may experience dyspnea on unaccustomed exertion.

Cardiac failure may be present in the resting state or may appear only with excessive stress. It is easily recognized in its later stages, when symptoms and signs due to pulmonary or systemic venous congestion, increased ventricular volume and diastolic pressure, and decreased cardiac output are present.

Cardiac failure may occur as a manifestation or complication of many types of heart disease. Not all patients with heart disease develop cardiac failure, however, and it is not known why some patients whose hearts have worked against increased loads for many years ultimately develop cardiac failure.

Cardiac failure may be 'forward' failure, as after myocardial infarction, in which the cardiac output is sharply reduced, or 'backward failure' when right ventricular failure follows left ventricular failure because of raised left atrial pressure and right ventricular dilatation. Congestive heart failure is diagnosed when systemic congestive phenomena (edema, enlarged and tender liver, raised venous pressure with pulsating neck veins) occur as a result of right ventricular failure, usually with tricuspid insufficiency. Left ventricular failure is diagnosed when pulmonary venous congestion follows left ventricular dilatation and increased left atrial pressure, manifested by dyspnea, orthopnea, paroxysmal nocturnal dyspnea and pulmonary edema. It is seen on a chest X-ray as pulmonary congestion.

In patients with heart disease, transient cardiac failure may be induced by any of the acute precipitating events (arrhythmias, respiratory infection, etc.). When the precipitating event subsides with time or is cured by appropriate treatment, the patient's cardiac status may return to its previous asymptomatic state. In these instances, it is more proper to speak of precipitation of reversible cardiac failure than spontaneous development of failure.

A definition of cardiac failure based not on symptoms but on objectively measured hemodynamic indices would be a useful clinical and research tool. For example, one may decide decide that cardiac failure is present when there is increased ventricular volume and ventricular end diastolic pressure and decreased cardiac output at rest or on exercise in patients with left ventricular disease due to any cause.

It should be obvious that the diagnosis of cardiac failure, like that of any other disease, depends upon its definition, which varies with different authorities. The distinction must be maintained between the presence of heart disease and the presence of cardiac failure, and the latter should be perceived as a continuum from (1) recognition of the presence of cardiac disease, to (2) a preclinical phase in which hemodynamic abnormalities but not symptoms may be present, and finally to (3) an overt clinical phase in which it is obvious to all that cardiac failure is present.

The heart fails ('decompensates') when various compensatory mechanism (cardiac hypertrophy, raised atrial pressure, ventricular dilatation, increased force of contraction are inadequate to maintain the function of a diseased heart whose work load has been increased.

As the compensatory mechanisms begin to falter, symptoms or hemodynamic indices of cardiac failure may not be obvious at rest but may be produced when the demands on the heart are increased by exercise, emotion, or precipitating factors. Depending upon what is being demanded, therefore, cardiac failure may be present when cardiac output is normal, increased (high output failure), or decreased.

Initially, either the left or, less commonly, the right ventricle may fail; ultimately, however, especially after salt and water retention occurs, combined left and right failure is the rule (congestive failure).

Left ventricular failure is most commonly due to hypertension, coronary heart disease, or valvular heart disease, usually aortic valvular disease; less common causes are mitral valve disease, congestive cardiomyopathies, hypertrophic cardiomyopathy, left-to-right shunts, and congenital heart lesions. Infective endocarditis may occur in a normal heart or may complicate other valvular disease and left ventricular failure may also occur. Cardiac failure may also occur in various connective tissue disorders, thyrotoxicosis, severe anemia, arteriovenous fistula, myocarditis, beriberi, and myocardial involvement by tumors or granulomas.

Isolated right ventricular failure is most commonly due to mitral stenosis with raised pulmonary vascular resistance, pulmonary parenchymal or vascular disease, or pulmonary valvular stenosis, less commonly, to tricuspid valvular disease or infective endocarditis involving the right side of the heart. Carcinoid disease involving the pulmonary or tricuspid valves is a rare cause. Systemic venous congestion follows, leading to congestive heart failure.

Factors Precipitating Failure

In at least half of cases, demonstrable precipitating disease or factors that increase the workload of the heart are present and these factors should be sought in every patient with cardiac failure. They include arrhythmias, respiratory infection, myocardial infarction, pulmonary embolism, rheumatic carditis, thyrotoxicosis, anemia excessive salt intake, corticosteroid administration, pregnancy, and excessive or rapid administration of parenteral fluids. Fever may aggravate failure (as in acute myocardial infarction) but does not cause it de novo.

Heart failure may occur in patients with normally functioning hearts that are subjected to excessive loads. The clearest example of this is systemic arteriovenous fistula. Even in otherwise healthy young people, a large fistula can produce heart failure, in older people, thyrotoxicosis, severe anemia, beriberi, or Paget's disease of bone may cause heart failure even though cardiac output is high.

Summary

The causes of ventricular failure can be summarized as follows:
1. Intrinsic myocardial disease, coronary heart disease, cardiomyopathy, infiltrative disease such as hemochromatosis, amyloidosis, sarcoidosis, and myocarditis.
2. Excess work load
   a. Increased resistance to ejection (pressure load): Hypertension, stenosis of aortic or pulmonary valves, hypertrophic cardiomyopathy.
   b. Increased stroke volume (volume load): Aortic insufficiency, mitral insufficiency, tricuspid insufficiency, congenital left-to-right shunts.
   c. Increased body demands ('high output failure'): Thyrotoxicosis, anemia, pregnancy, arteriovenous fistula.

■ CLINICAL FINDINGS

When a patient with any type of heart disease congenital, valvular, hypertensive, coronary, metabolic, etc. develops symptoms and signs of cardiac failure, the findings are usually not specific for any particular etiologic category.

Symptoms and signs of pulmonary or systemic venous congestion, increased cardiac volume, and diastolic pressure combined with decreased cardiac output, raised venous pressure, and evidences of salt and water retention clearly indicate that cardiac failure has occurred. In patients with congenital heart disease, pulmonary heart disease, endocarditis involving the valves on the right side, primary pulmonary hypertension, or obstructive diseases of the lungs, raised venous pressure, enlarged tender liver, and systemic edema indicate that cardiac disease has progressed to right sided congestive failure. This is also true when pulmonary hypertension complicates mitral stenosis and right heart failure and tricuspid regurgitation follow. Right heart failure occurs most commonly as a sequel to left heart failure. Right heart failure is the rule in congenital heart disease, although there is a variety of congenital lesions such as patent ducts arteriosus, coarctation of the aorta, ventricular septal defect, and tricuspid atresia in which the excess load is on the left ventricle, which may ultimately fail. These conditions are all discussed in greater detail elsewhere in this book.

The manifestations of congestive heart failure vary depending on the cause, on the nature of the failure (acute or chronic), and on the location of primary load (left ventricle, right ventricle, or both).

Left Ventricular Failure

Before symptoms of left ventricular failure develop, the patient will show evidence of the primary disease (unless failure follows acute myocardial infarction), such as hypertension or aortic stenosis, as well as physical signs of left ventricular hypertrophy and other compensatory changes in the left ventricle. When the compensatory mechanism fail, the left ventricular end-diastolic pressure rises, and this increased pressure is transmitted to the left atrium and to the pulmonary veins, resulting in pulmonary venous congestion which is recognized hemodynamically by a rise in pulmonary capillary wedge pressure. Depending upon the acuteness and magnitude of the rise in pressure in the pulmonary capillaries, transudation of fluid into the tissue spaces occurs when the pulmonary capillary wedge pressure exceeds the combination of the oncotic pressure of serum and tissue pressure. If the removal of fluid from the tissue spaces via the lymphatics is incomplete, fluid appears in the alveoli, causing more acute symptoms.

Symptoms

1. **Dyspnea**: Both by reflex action and by increased work of breathing, the increased fluid in the tissue spaces causes dyspnea, at first on effort and then at rest. The work of breathing is greater because of the increased stiffness of the lungs, and the patient is aware of difficulty in breathing. Transudation of fluid into the alveoli superimposes cough on dyspnea of effort and this combination is suggestive of left ventricular failure. The symptoms are usually progressive, and the earliest manifestation is shortness of breath on exertion that previously caused no difficulty. As pulmonary engorgement progresses, less and less activity brings on dyspnea and cough, until both are present even when the patient is at rest.

2. **Orthopnea:** Shortness of breath in recumbency, which is promptly relieved by propping up the head or trunk, is precipitated by the increase in pulmonary engorgement that occurs in the recumbent position. When the pulmonary blood volume is thus increased, the patient characteristically goes to sleep without difficulty but awakens several hours later with dyspnea (paroxysmal nocturnal dyspnea). The mechanism is believed to be increased pulmonary blood volume associated with recumbency and the autotransfusion of fluid accumulated in the lower half of the body during upright posture when the blood is returned to the heart. The enhanced venous return (Frank-Starling mechanism) results in greater force

of contraction to restore the status quo; when ventricular performance is on or near the descending limb of the Frank-Starling curve, increased contractility cannot compensate for the greater venous return.

3. **Paroxysmal nocturnal dyspnea:** Paroxysmal nocturnal dyspnea with cough usually develops in a setting of progressive dyspnea on exertion and orthopnea, but it may appear at any time and may be the first manifestation of left ventricular failure in severe hypertension, aortic stenosis or insufficiency, or myocardial infarction. It also occurs in patients with tight mitral stenosis, but in this condition, it is due to pulmonary venous congestion from obstruction at the mitral valve rather than left ventricular failure. Paroxysmal nocturnal dyspnea or cough is an exaggerated form of orthopnea and may be associated with inspiratory and expiratory wheezing from bronchospasm (so-called cardiac asthma). Depending upon the amount of fluid that accumulates in the lungs. The patient with paroxysmal nocturnal dyspnea may awaken with dyspnea that lasts only a few minutes and is relieved by sitting or standing or the dyspnea may progress rapidly into an alarming episode of pulmonary edema.

4. **Acute pulmonary edema:** Acute pulmonary edema resulting from gross transudation of fluid into the alveoli from the rapidly rising pulmonary capillary pressure causes the patient to sit up in bed gasping for breath; the patient is also cold, pale, anxious, sweating profusely, and prevented by air hunger from finishing a sentence. The patient may become cyanotic, cough up frothy white or pink sputum and be fearful of imminent death. Patients may ignore progressive dyspnea on exertion, but they rarely ignore acute pulmonary edema. Most attacks subside gradually in 1–3 hours, possibly because of the upright position as well as the progressive decrease in cardiac output. In some instances, the left ventricle rapidly weakens, leading to shock and death. Left atrial pressure has been shown to rise to 50 or 60 mm Hg when measured during episodes of pulmonary edema.

Heroin administration is one of the common causes of pulmonary edema, the mechanism of action is presumably the increased capillary permeability. This results in arterial hypoxemia and acidosis, which can be quite marked. The arterial PO_2 is usually less than 40 mm Hg in the presence of pulmonary edema, and the pH hovers around 7.15.

5. **Interpretation of dyspnea:** When dyspnea on exertion is the only symptom, its interpretation is often difficult, especially when the patient is obese and in poor physical condition.

   a. Patients in poor physical condition almost never have orthopnea or paroxysmal nocturnal dyspnea, and the dyspnea is rarely progressive over a short period of time as it is when left ventricular failure develops in aortic stenosis or coronary disease.

   b. Pulmonary causes of dyspnea such as chronic bronchitis, pulmonary fibrosis, and asthmatic bronchitis are more difficult to differentiate because the wheezing of left ventricular failure due to bronchospasm may simulate that of asthma. However, the patient with chronic lung disease usually gives a history of smoking, longstanding cough, or sputum production and frequent episodes of purulent bronchitis in winter. Cough is often present in the absence of dyspnea.

   c. Moderate to severe anemia may also produce exertional dyspnea.

   d. Advanced age, debility, extreme obesity, ascites from any cause, abdominal distention from gastrointestinal disease, or advanced stages of pregnancy may produce orthopnea in the absence of heart disease.

e. **Neurocirculatory asthenia:** Patients with neurocirculatory asthenia or anxiety states with psychophysiologic cardiovascular reactions may suffer from sighing respirations simulating dyspnea. This syndrome is more frequent in wartime, though it also occurs in civilian life. So-called soldier's heart is associated with fatigue, chest pain, and palpitations and is induced by activities related to being a member of the armed forces unwillingly and under unpleasant circumstance.

6. **Fatigue:** Exertional fatigue and weakness due to reduced cardiac output are late symptoms and disappear promptly with rest. Severe fatigue rather than dyspnea is the chief complaint of patients with mitral stenosis who have developed pulmonary hypertension and low cardiac output.

7. **Nocturia as a symptom of edema:** Nocturia may represent excretion of edema fluid accumulated during the day and increased renal perfusion in the recumbent position, it reflects the decreased work of the heart at rest and often the effects of diuretics given during the day. It may also be due to noncardiac causes.

Signs

Evidence of the primary disease responsible for the failure, e.g. hypertension or aortic stenosis, is usually present. In some instances of severe failure due to aortic stenosis, the murmur may be absent or difficult to hear because of the decreased velocity of ejection and reduced cardiac output.

Evidence of so-called primary disease is at times misleading. For example, because of the compensatory systemic vasoconstriction that occurs in any condition with reduced cardiac output via the baroreceptor mechanism, blood pressure may be modestly raised in patients with cardiac failure due to any cause; one should

therefore be cautious in defining the disease as hypertensive heart failure unless the blood pressure remains elevated after the failure is relieved by treatment.

Left ventricular failure may occur acutely with fluid overload, as may happen with too rapid infusion of large amounts of blood or saline in patients with minimal evidence of left ventricular failure prior to the infusion. Ventricular or atrial arrhythmias associated with a rapid ventricular rate, severe anemia, acute leukemia or abrupt slowing of the ventricular rate, as in atrioventricular block, may abruptly result in left ventricular failure. Unaccustomed severe exertion, as in severe aortic stenosis, may cause acute left ventricular failure and may be the first manifestation of failure in patients with aortic stenosis. Drugs such as propranolol that have a negative inotropic effect may rapidly cause left ventricular failure by removing sympathetic drive to the heart and should be used with caution in patients with incipient left ventricular failure.

1. **Enlargement of heart:** In the presence of symptoms of cardiac failure, hypertrophy or dilatation of the left ventricle is usually found on examination and confirmed by evidence of left ventricular hypertrophy on the ECG and left ventricular enlargement on the X-ray or echocardiogram.

2. **Ventricular heave:** The best clinical sign of left ventricular hypertrophy is a left ventricular heave at the apex of the heart. The heave is a localized, sustained, systolic outward motion of the left ventiruclar impulse that differs from the hyperdynamic left ventricular impulse of exertion, anxiety, or regurgitant valve disease and from the right ventricular heave of right ventricular hypertrophy. The latter is more diffuse, is felt over the center of the chest, and causes apical retraction rather than a lift during systole.

3. **Third heart sound:** When there is increased left ventricular volume, an exaggerated third heart sound is often heard as ventricular filling occurs during the rapid inflow phase.

4. **Fourth heart sound:** Decreased compliance of the left ventricle with resultant hypertrophy of the left atrium causes a fourth heart sound or atrial gallop which may be felt or seen and is also manifested by a large a wave in jugular venous pulse or in the apex cardiogram.

5. **Rales:** Rales in the lungs may be absent at rest and even early in the episode of nocturnal dyspnea, when transudation occurs into the tissue spaces and not into the alveoli. Later, however, when alveolar fluid appears, the rales are loud and generalized frothy, bubbling fluid may be obvious all over the lungs. Pleural effusion may occur.

6. **Cheyne-Stokes respiration:** Cheyne Stokes-respiration is commonly seen in advanced cardiac failure. A typical illustration of the beneficial effects of aminophylline can be seen. Following administration of intravenous aminophylline, there is a fall in PCO_2, progressive decrease in the duration of the apneic period until the respirations are normal, and an increase in minute volume respiration.

7. **Tachycardia:** As the stroke volume decreases, tachycardia compensates to increase the minute cardiac output; it is usually present in cardiac failure.

8. **Pulsus alternans.**

Right Ventricular Failure

Right ventricular failure is usually secondary to chronic left ventricular failure but may occur alone. The most common causes of right ventricular failure are tight mitral stenosis with pulmonary hypertension, pulmonary valve stenosis, cor pulmonale from chronic lung disease, primary pulmonary hypertension with tricuspid insufficiency and other congenital diseases such as Eisenmenger's complex and pulmonary hypertensive ventricular or atrial septal defects. Tricuspid valve disease may produce the same systemic venous congestion, but like mitral stenosis, the congestion is due to obstruction at the tricuspid valve and not to right ventricular failure unless there is an associated obstruction higher up, such as mitral stenosis. Rare cause is involvement of the pulmonary and tricuspid valves from carcinoid or infective endocarditis. Right ventricular infarction is a somewhat more common cause.

Symptoms

The dominant symptoms of right ventricular failure are those of systemic venous congestion in contrast to left ventricular failure, in which symptoms of pulmonary venous congestion predominate. Pulmonary symptoms are rare unless there is associated left ventricular failure or unless right ventricular failure is due to chronic lung disease. Paroxysmal nocturnal dyspnea is uncommon.

1. **Fatigue:** The patient may complain of fatigue as cardiac output is reduced.

2. **Dependent edema:** Edema of the ankles may occur when the patient is up and about; edema of the sacrum, flanks, and thighs when in bed.

3. **Liver engorgement:** If right ventricular failure occurs rapidly, as when atrial fibrillation develops in tight mitral stenosis, congestion of the liver with distension of its capsule may result, causing right upper quadrant pain, which has often been confused with that of cholecystitis or other abdominal disease.

4. **Anorexia and bloating:** Hepatic and visceral engorgement secondary to the raised venous pressure may cause anorexia, bloating, and other nonspecific gastrointestinal symptoms.

Signs

Evidence of the underlying disease is usually found when specifically sought although special investigations may be necessary.

1. **Right ventricular hypertrophy:** In primary right ventricular failure, right ventricular hypertrophy can be diagnosed on the basis of right ventricular heave and right atrial gallop rhythm by auscultation.

2. **Right ventricular heave:** A right ventricular heave over the lower central chest, pulsation of the pulmonary arteries if there is increased pulmonary blood flow, right atrial gallop rhythm, a loud pulmonary second sound at the base of the heart, and increased jugular venous pressure with systolic pulsations of tricuspid insufficiency are usually present.

3. **Right atrial gallop:** A right S3 is often heard, especially when right ventricular failure is due to increased resistance to right ventricular outflow, as in pulmonary stenosis or pulmonary hypertension.

4. **Murmurs:** If the underlying disease is congenital or valvular, characteristic murmurs will be heard, although in some patients with Eisenmenger's syndrome with severe pulmonary hypertension and a balanced shunt flow no murmurs may be heard—as is true also of primary pulmonary hypertension and chronic lung disease.

5. **Chronic pulmonary signs:** If right ventricular failure is secondary to chronic lung disease, there will be evidence of decreased distensibility of the lungs, rales, rhonchi, wheezes, and signs of chronic bronchitis.

6. **Jugular pulse:** Careful inspection of the jugular venous pulse will not only demonstrate the pulsating systolic wave of tricuspid insufficiency (which may also be palpated over the liver, with systolic expansion of the liver). There may also be prominent presystolic a waves when there is decreased compliance of the right ventricle and raised right atrial pressure, a waves are also prominent in pulmonary stenosis with right ventricular failure and in tricuspid stenosis. The venous pressure rises further when right upper quadrant pressure is exerted by the physician, and the right atrial pressure may be raised as much as 5 mm Hg by this maneuver (hepatojugular reflux). The systolic jugular venous pulse of tricuspid insufficiency is often associated with a pansystolic murmur over the xiphoid, often accentuated by inspiration and associated with a right atrial gallop, which is also louder on inspiration.

7. **Pulmonary second sound:** The pulmonary second sound is accentuated if there is pulmonary hypertension but may be absent in severe pulmonary stenosis and fainter, with a wider split from A2, if pulmonary stenosis is mild to moderate.

8. **Pitting edema:** Pitting edema of the ankles, lower extremities, and back is found in established right ventricular failure.

9. **Ascites:** Initially, the dependent edema caused by right heart failure usually subsides overnight. Eventually, it fails to subside with initial bed rest and may even increase during recumbency. Ascites is rarely prominent unless right ventricular failure has been neglected or if obstructive lesions such as constrictive pericarditis, tricuspid stenosis, or cardiac tamponade are present. In these instances, the jugular venous pressure is raised but there is no clinical evidence of tricuspid insufficiency, in fact, the dominant wave seen in the neck may be a prominently descent.

10. **Hydrothorax (pleural effusion) Hydrothorax:** is common in congestive heart failure, occurring in about a third of severe cases. It is more common in right than in left ventricular failure and more apt to occur in the right pleural space than in the left; bilateral hydrothorax is less common. Some authorities believe that isolated left hydrothorax should make one consider other conditions such as pulmonary infarction, but well documented isolated left hydrothorax has often been reported. Fluid may accumulate in any serous cavity (e.g. the pericardial and peritoneal cavities the latter more apt to result from tricuspid stenosis of constrictive pericarditis). Rapid changes in the heart shadow should make one think of pericardial effusion rather than shrinkage of cardiac enlargement.

High Output Failure

Arteriovenous fistula is an uncommon cause of heart failure and may be congenital or acquired. The congenital variety may be due to congenital arteriovenous angioma, often involving a limb. Acquired fistulas are due to trauma (including surgical trauma), usually involving the larger arteries of the limbs. They may be visceral (e.g. following nephrectomy) or musculoskeletal (e.g. after laminectomy). The condition may be insidious, and the fistula may not be clinically obvious.

Arteriovenous fistulas are created surgically in patients with renal disease in order to facilitate hemodialysis. Although such arteriovenous shunts are well tolerated by patients with normal hearts, they may cause heart failure in older patients with associated heart lesions. In high output failure due to other causes such as severe anemia, Paget's disease of bone, thyrotoxicosis, or beriberi, the factor responsible for the failure is usually less obvious.

Symptoms

Dyspnea on exertion, edema of the ankles, and fatigue are indistinguishable from the same symptoms occurring the other patients with heart failure.

Signs

It is the physical signs of high output failure that provide the clue to diagnosis. The cardinal sign in tachycardia that is disproportionate to the degree of failure and associated with a hyperdynamic cardiac impulse and clinical evidence of cardiac enlargement. Venous pressure is often elevated, and the pulse pressure is widened. A systolic ejection murmur may be heard at the base, resulting from increased stroke volume. If the patient has an arteriovenous aneurysm in a limb, where it can be occluded, it is useful to determine whether occlusion of the fistula has any effect on heart rate. In large fistulas, occlusion increases peripheral resistance, raises systemic arterial

pressure, and causes a reflex bradycardia via the baroreceptor, reflexes (Branham's sign). If this sign is positive, the fistula is large enough to be a potential cause of heart failure.

Acute Heart Failure

When cardiac failure is acute, the clinical picture is different in different disorders and will be described in the respective sections dealing with specific causes of acute failure. For example, when the chordae of the mitral valve rupture, acute to subacute pulmonary venous congestion occurs, with rapid development of mitral regurgitation and left ventricular failure. However, the left atrium is smaller, sinus rhythm is the rule, and the clinical picture differs from that of chronic mitral regurgitation.

Differential Diagnosis

Cardiac failure must be distinguished from all conditions associated with dyspnea, cough, pulmonary venous congestion, venous pressure elevation, decreased cardiac output, cardiac enlargement, or peripheral edema. These clinical findings occur in a wide variety of conditions that can be conveniently discussed in groups, as in the following paragraphs.

Noncardiac and Nonthoracic Conditions Simulating Cardiac Failure

Examples include the dyspnea and fatigue of obesity, of sedentary individuals, and of emotional states with hyperventilation, and the edema that occurs as a result of thrombophlebitis or prolonged sitting in people with varicose veins. In these conditions, there are usually no objective signs of heart disease such as significant murmurs, friction rub, gallop rhythm, cardiac enlargement, or raised venous pressure. Cardiac diagnostic procedures noninvasive or invasive reveal no abnormalities of the cardiovascular system. At times, these symptoms and signs from non-cardiac causes occur in patients with known cardiac disease. As indicted in the introductory paragraphs, the presence of cardiac disease does not imply that all of the patient's symptoms and signs are due to cardiac failure.

Cardiac failure must be diagnosed on the basis of symptoms and signs.

Lung Disease and Acute Respiratory Tract infections Presenting with Respiratory Symptoms

Right heart failure may occur in chronic lung disease (cor pulmonale), but many patients with chronic lung disease, chronic bronchitis, emphysema, etc. have dyspnea and cough for many years without abnormality of the heart. Patients with acute respiratory symptoms may have acute infections of the bronchi or lungs associated with fever and other symptoms and signs of acute illness. The differential diagnosis, including clinical and pulmonary function studies. Most helpful in chronic lung disease in the long history of chronic cough and sputum production, dyspnea and wheezing, combined with clinical findings of poor lung expansion and chronic wheezes and rales. A history of cigarette smoking or of repeated respiratory infections in the absence of cardiac enlargement, gallop rhythm, ventricular heaves, or raised venous pressure is most helpful. Venous pressure becomes elevated when cardiac failure complicates chronic lung disease, but pulmonary symptoms are present for many years without this objective finding. Pulmonary function studies aid in the diagnosis of specific chronic lung diseases, and hemodynamic studies reveal increases of pressure in the pulmonary artery and the right heart with no abnormality in the left heart. When the two conditions coexist, the differentiation may be difficult.

Massive Pulmonary Embolism

Pulmonary embolism may produce symptoms similar to those of cardiac failure, or acute right ventricular failure may follow; (1) massive pulmonary embolism with the development of acute pulmonary infarction as noted on chest X-ray or (2) pulmonary hypertension associated with signs of acute right ventricular overload, with physical signs of pulmonary hypertension and evidence on the ECG of right ventricular dilatation rather than systemic venous congestion (Sokolow, 1940). More precise diagnosis is provided by the combination of chest X-ray, pulmonary radioisotope scan, and pulmonary angiography.

Diseases of the Pericardium and Myocardium

The most important distinguishing feature is raised left ventricular filling pressure relative to the right side, indicating that the disease is due to congestive cardiomyopathy with cardiac failure. Echocardiography is helpful in recognizing and quantifying the presence of pericardial effusion, which may not be suspected clinically, although findings of pericarditis such as pericardial friction rub can be diagnostic.

Chapter 3

Congenital Heart Disease

INTRODUCTION

Congenital heart disease need not manifest or produce symptoms/signs at birth. Congenital heart disease represents the largest share of pediatric cardiologic practice. Increasing emphasis has been placed on investigation and treatment of younger patients with congenital heart lesions. Neonatal cardiology, which differs significantly from adult cardiology, is a subject of great current interest. Although it is reasonable to equate congenital heart disease in older children (6 years and over) with that seen in adults, it is not possible to devise a single description of the characteristics of congenital heart disease encompassing neonatal, infant, and adult disease. This chapter is confined to the clinical picture of congenital lesions as seen in adults and older children and does not purport to describe congenital heart disease as seen in infants.

SURGICALLY MODIFIED DISEASE

Because of increasing longevity, more patients are being seen in adult life who have had corrective or palliative surgery for congenital lesions in infancy or childhood. In many of these patients, the disease has been surgically modified, creating new unnatural conditions that merit clinical description. The best example is the effect on congenital disease of an earlier palliative surgical procedure (Blalock's operation) for relief of Fallot's tetralogy. Many patients with Fallot's tetralogy now seen as adults have had a palliative operation, and the long-term effects on the clinical status of the patient are clearly important.

CLASSIFICATION OF CONGENITAL HEART DISEASE

There is no satisfactory classification of congenital heart disease. A classification based on embryologic studies is too comprehensive for use in adult patients because most individuals with extensive defects do not survive. The following clinical classification, based on that of Wood, gives an indication of the relative frequency with which the various lesions are encountered **after puberty**.

Without Shunt

1. Right-sided

Pulmonary stenosis	25%
Ebstein's malformation	Rare

2. Left-sided Coarctation of the aorta — 5%

With Shunt

1. Acyanotic (Left to Right)

Atrial septal defect	30%
Patent ductus arteriosus	7%
Ventricular septal defect	9%

2. Cyanotic (Right to Left/ bidirectional)

Tetralogy of Fallot	10%
Eisenmenger's syndrome	7%
Ebsetin's malformation	Rare
Transposition of great vessels	Rare
Truncus arteriosus	Rare
Tricuspid atresia	Rare

This classification omits isolated valvular lesions such as aortic stenosis and congenital mitral lesions in which the cause cannot always be identified with certainty. The various lesions in combination, e.g. atrial septal defect with pulmonary stenosis and atrial plus ventricular septal defect can be mentioned.

ATRIAL SEPTAL DEFECT

Cardinal Features and Pathogenesis

The essential feature of atrial septal defect is a left-to-right shunt of arterialized blood into the right atrium that produces a high tricuspid flow and increased blood flow to the lungs, with a normal pulmonary arterial pressure. The severity of the lesion depends primarily on the size of the defect, which in turn limits the size of the shunt. The size of the defect is not the sole determinant of the severity of the lesions, however, as can be seen from the natural history of the condition. Atrial septal defect is often not diagnosed in infancy or childhood. At birth, the right and left ventricles are equal in size and thickness in normal infants, and right-to-left shunt in a patient foramen ovale can normally occur. Whenever an atrial septal defect is present, however, left-to-right shunting is minimal at birth. With the normal decrease in pulmonary vascular resistance that follows birth, the right ventricle becomes more complaint. It then fills more readily than the left ventricle, and as a result, left-to-right shunting becomes apparent. Most atrial septal defects are large enough (2 × 2 cm or more) to equalize pressure between the right and the left atrium. Thus, the magnitude of the left-to-right shunt depends mainly on the filling characteristics of the right and left ventricles. In most cases (85%), in which the diagnosis can be made, the left-to-right shunt is at least equal to the left ventricular output, so that pulmonary flow is more than twice systemic flow. The pulmonary circulation reading accepts the increased pulmonary flow, so that pulmonary arterial pressure is usually low. The presence of anomalous venous drainage does not affect the clinical picture, but the presence of associated mitral or tricuspid incompetence or a complete endocardial cushion defect makes the lesion more severe.

The increase in flow involves both atria, the right ventricle, and the pulmonary circulation, but not the left ventricle or the aorta in uncomplicated cases. The extra load on the heart is a pure 'flow load' and is well tolerated for many years. Since the magnitude of the left-to-right shunt depends on the relative diastolic compliances of the two ventricles, the shunt is not fixed. Any factor that increases the load on the left ventricle tends to decrease its compliance and increase the left-to-right shunt. Conversely, anything that increases the assistance of right ventricular emptying decreases the shunt and tends to reverse it.

Clinical Findings

Symptoms and Signs

Atrial septal defect is difficult to diagnose, and the examiner must maintain a high index of suspicion if all cases are to be recognized and treated surgically.

a. About half of patients with atrial septal defect are asymptomatic when the diagnosis is made. Symptoms develop in 60% of patients by age 30. This indicates that the lesion is often noted in early adult life, either on routine physical examination or (more often) on a chest X-ray. The commonest presenting symptom is dyspnea on exertion (65%), followed by palpitations due to atrial arrhythmia (20%), and chest pain, which is usually not angina in nature. A spurious past history of rheumatic fever may be present (5%). Children with left-to-right shunts are prone to develop bronchitis and other lung infections. In about 20% of adult cases, the diagnosis of atrial septal defect presents some difficulty, either because the patient is middle aged and the possibility of a congenital lesion is not considered or because the clinical picture is atypical. In about half of these cases, the patient is in right heart failure when first seen, in such cases, edema and ascites tend to be more prominent than dyspnea.

i.   Patients with Marfan's syndrome, a congenital mesodermal abnormality associated with cystic medial necrosis of the aorta and ectopia lentis, may have atrial septal defect. Patients with other skeletal abnormalities may also have the lesion (e.g. Ehlers-Danlos syndrome), and atrial septal defect is said to occur in tall, thin persons with long spidery fingers (arachnodactyly) and a high-arched palate, but these appearances are not of diagnostic value.

ii. **Cardiac signs:** The physical signs depend on the magnitude of pulmonary blood flow. Increased right ventricular stroke volume produces a hyperdynamic right ventricular impulse with a visible and palpable pulse over the pulmonary artery in the second or third left intercostals space. A pulmonary systolic ejection murmur is almost always present because of increased flow through the pulmonary valve, but the murmur is often slight. The first heart sound is often loud because the tricuspid valve closes from a wide open position with right ventricular systole. There is relative tricuspid stenosis in patients with atrial septal defect because the diastolic flow across the tricuspid valve is usually twice the normal value or more. In addition to the loud tricuspid first sound, there is often a right sided third sound and a tricuspid diastolic murmur that becomes louder during inspiration.

Second heart sound: The second heart sound is widely split in patients with atrial septal defect. The normal widening of the split with inspiration does not occur, and the failure of the second sound to become single on expiration

(fixed split) is an important clue to the presence of the lesion. These findings are caused by the combination of delayed activation of the right ventricle and prolonged ejection time associated with increased right ventricular stroke volume. Inspiration has little effect on the condition because only a relatively small increase in the already large flow occurs through the pulmonary valve upon inspiration.

iii. **Ostium primum defects:** In patients with ostium primum defects there may also be a hyperdynamic left ventricular impuse and a pansystolic apical murmur if mitral incompetence in present. Tricuspid incompetence is a defect that also occurs with ostium primum defects, giving a pansystolic murmur that is best heard at the left lower sternal border. Incompetence of the atrioventricular valves can also occur in ostium secundum defects, especially when heart failure develops.

iv. **Pulse:** The pulse is of small amplitude, and the venous pressure is normal. Atrial fibrillation commonly develops after age 40, and other varieties of atrial arrhythmia are also seen.

Differential Diagnosis

A. **Rheumatic Heart Disease:** Atrial septal defect is likely to be misdiagnosed as rheumatic mitral valve disease with mixed mitral stenosis and incompetence. The combination of cardiac enlargement, systolic and diastolic murmurs arising at the atrioventricular valve and atrial fibrillation in a middle-aged woman can easily be mistaken for a rheumatic lesion, and pulmonary plethora due to increased blood flow can be confused in the chest X-ray with pulmonary congestion. If there is no rsR pattern on the ECG, the possibility of a congenital lesion may not be considered until cardiac catheterization reveals a high pulmonary arterial oxygen saturation. The presence of a large heart with only mild symptoms and the patient's ability to easily tolerate the onset of atrial fibrillation should suggest the possibility of an atrial defect. A large pulmonary artery and right atrium, combined with a small aorta and small left atrium on the chest X-ray, should suggest a possible diagnosis of atrial septal defect.

B. Other Lesions: Small atrial septal defects may be confused with a normal heart picture, especially is the presence of pectus excavatum, which tends to cause systolic and even diastolic murmurs and to make the heart look large on posteroanterior view. Idiopathic dilatation of the pulmonary artery may also lead to confusion. It causes a systolic ejection murmur a widely split second heart sound, and a large main pulmonary artery on the chest X-ray, and it is often associated with an rsR pattern in lead V1 of the ECG. Cardiac catheterization must always be accurate enough to provide a correct diagnosis.

Complications

A. **Pulmonary Vascular Disease:** Pulmonary vascular disease is the most important complication of atrial septal defect. In patients with ostium secundum defects, it is always acquired rather than congenital. In patients with ostium primum or sinus venous defects with anomalous venous drainage, the congenital form of pulmonary hypertension occurs, in which a raised pulmonary vascular resistance is present in infancy or childhood and does not develop in later life. In patients with acquired pulmonary hypertension, the heart is large, the patient is usually over age 20, and pulmonary hypertension is progressive. Acquired pulmonary hypertension is due to the long-term effects of increased pulmonary blood flow on the pulmonary vascular bed,

and pulmonary thromboembolism may initiate or aggravate the condition, especially in pregnancy. The incidence of this form of pulmonary hypertension, sometimes called acquired Eisenmerger's syndrome, is decreasing with earlier and more accurate diagnosis of congenital heart disease, but it still occurs in about 10% of cases. This complication is not inevitable, and patients with atrial septal defect who have been recatheterized after an interval of up to 20 years usually show no significant increase in pulmonary vascular resistance.

1. **Symptoms and signs of pulmonary vascular disease:** Increased dyspnea or cyanosis on exertion and intolerance of altitude are the commonest presenting symptoms. The patient may develop cyanosis and clubbing of the fingers, and polycythemia and increase in hematocrit are almost invariably found. There is usually a large a wave in the jugular venous pulse, and the heart is almost always greatly enlarged, with a prominent right ventricular heave. A pulmonary ejection click and a loud pulmonary valve closure sound are heard. The ECG shows right ventricular hypertrophy and often atrial fibrillation. Chest X-ray confirms cardiac enlargement and usually shows marked enlargement of the central pulmonary arteries. There is a progressive increase in the heart size and also in the size of the pulmonary arteries.

2. **Cardiac catheterization:** Cardiac catheterization shows pulmonary arterial hypertension and a pulmonary blood flow that is normal or only slightly increased. Right-to-left shunting may be present at rest, with an arterial saturation of 85–95%, or desaturation may develop during exercise. Accurate measurement of pulmonary vascular resistance, plus study of the effects of vasodilator drugs such as tolazoline (Priscoline) or

acetylcholine plus oxygen breathing, is needed to decide whether surgery is warranted. Closure of the defect is likely to be successful when the upper level of pulmonary vascular resistance does not exceed 7.5 mm Hg/L/min. The magnitude of the left-to-right shunt is a factor of almost equal importance. If the pulmonary blood flow is increased, closing the defect can reduce the load on pulmonary circulation and reverse or half the progress of pulmonary vascular disease. Surgery in advanced cases has a high mortality rate, and the results are poor because the 'safety valve' of an actual or potential right-to-left shunt is removed.

B. Heart Failure: Heart failure is the other, almost equally important complication of atrial septal defect. It is usually seen in association with atrial fibrillation and is directly related to the age of the patient and the presence of a lesion interfering with filling of the left ventricle. The natural course of atrial septal defect that is not surgically treated, heart failure probably occurs with almost the same frequency as shunt reversal due to pulmonary hypertension. The exact mechanism of the congestive heart failure is not clear.

i. It is possible that mechanical factors play a part, because the enlarged right ventricle displaces the left ventricular posteriorly. This abnormal position of the left ventricle, suggests that bulging of the right ventricle into the left interferes with filling. Left ventricular filling is apparently compromised by deterioration in left ventricular function secondary to systemic hypertension, coronary arterial disease, or advancing age. When the left ventricle does not fill properly, its compliance decreases and its diastolic pressure rises. As left atrial pressure tends to increase the magnitude of the left-to-right shunt increases and

loads the right heart. Atrial fibrillation and tricuspid incompetence tend to aggravate the situation, and right heart failure with edema, hepatomegaly, and raised jugular pressure follows. The right and left atrial pressures are the same if the defect is large, and values as high as 15–20 mm Hg are common. These levels are not sufficient to cause serious pulmonary congestion but are enough to produce significant right-sided congestion. The response to treatment with digitalis and diuretics is good, and the prognosis in surgical closure of the defect is much better than was formerly thought.

C. Atrial Arrhythmias: Atrial fibrillation and other atrial arrhythmias are almost inevitable, especially atrial fibrillation after age 40 in the absence of surgical treatment. These arrhythmias are also related to the severity of the lesion and are less common in patients with small shunts. Restoration of sinus rhythm should be done unless arrhythmia is well tolerated.

D. Other Complications: Infective endocarditis is rare in atrial septal defect. Patients with ostium primum defects are more prone to develop this complication than are those with other atrial septal defects, presumably because of valvular involvement. Mitral valve disease is an associated lesion rather than a complication. The lesion is usually mild but tends to readily produce congestive heart failure by reducing systemic flow and increasing the left-to-right shunt.

■ PULMONARY STENOSIS

Cardinal Features

Pulmonary stenosis includes a number of conditions in which blood flow from the right heart to the lungs is obstructed.

The cardinal features include reduction in pulmonary blood flow, right ventricular hypertrophy, and a murmur at the site of obstruction. Among the variable factors that may be operating, the severity of obstruction influences the pulmonary blood flow and the extent of hypertrophy,. Other factors are the site of obstruction (valvular, infundibular, or in the pulmonary artery) and the patency of the foramen ovale, which determines the presence of reversed interatrial shunt.

Various combinations of obstruction lesions are possible, and the severity of the obstruction varies. The principal load is on the right ventricle. The pulmonary artery is often dilated at the point at which the jet of blood passing through the narrowed valve impinges on the artery (poststenotic dilatation). In severe cases, a patent foramen ovale may permit right-to-left shunting at the atrial level. Pulmonary stenosis is the second most common form of congenital heart disease to adults mainly because the category includes patients with hemodynamically insignificant lesions. Two-thirds of adult cases are mild, and many could be classified as examples of idiopathic dilatation of the pulmonary artery. The spectrum of cases, wide both because of differences in severity and because of varying sites of obstruction.

Pulmonary stenosis is more common in women than in men and is well tolerated in all but its severest forms. In mild cases the right ventricular systolic pressure is less than 50 mm Hg and the gradient across the stenosis is 20 or 30 mm Hg at rest. In moderate cases, the right ventricular systolic pressure is in the range of 50–100 mm Hg, with a gradient of up to 80 mm Hg. In severe cases, the diagnosis is usually made in childhood, and severe cases with right ventricular pressures at or above systemic level are rarely seen in adults.

Clinical Findings

Symptoms and Signs

Hemodynamically insignificant or mild pulmonary stenosis does not cause significant symptoms. If a murmur has been detected, the patient may be abnormally aware of the heart and develop noncardiac pain.

1. **Dyspnea:** Dyspnea is the commonest presenting symptom in patients with moderate or severe pulmonary stenosis. Its origin is obscure, and the conventional explanation of cardiac dyspnea pulmonary congestion and reduced lung compliance is not applicable. Patients with pulmonary stenosis tend to hyperventilate during exercise and inadequate perfusion of the exercising muscles is thought in provoke reflex ventilator stimulation.

2. **Dizziness and faintness on exertion, palpitation and chest pain:** These may rarely be the presenting symptoms in severe cases of pulmonary stenosis. The chest pain may be indistinguishable from that of angina of effort, and the fainting attacks are similar to the syncope on unaccustomed effort that occurs in patients with severe aortic stenosis.

3. **Right heart failure:** Right heart failure often occurs in early adult life in severe cases, and if the patient has not been seen previously, the diagnosis may be difficult when the patient presents in right heart failure with as extremely low cardiac output and little or no murmur.

The pulse is of small amplitude and there is a giant a wave in the jugular venous pulse in severe cases. A right ventricular substernal heave is felt in moderate and severe cases.

A systolic murmur is always present except in moribund patients. In cases of valvular stenosis, the duration of the murmur is a function of the severity of the lesion. In mild cases of valvular stenosis, the murmur is short and diamond shaped on the tracing. It is preceded by an ejection click. If the obstruction is infundibular, the murmur is longer and more like the pansystolic murmur of ventricular septal defect. In pulmonary artery stenosis, the murmur peaks later and resembles the murmur of coarctation of the aorta. The loudness and timing of the pulmonary valve closure sound are valuable clues to the severity of valvular stenotic lesions. In mild cases, the second sound is normally or widely split, and the split moves normally with respiration. In moderately severe lesions, the pulmonary closure sound is delayed occurring up to 0.1 second after aortic closure. It is also diminished in intensity because pulmonary blood flow tends to be low, but it still moves with inspiration. In severe cases, the pulmonary valve closure sound is inaudible, and even aortic closure may not be heard because the sound is buried in the long pulmonary systolic murmur which results from prolonged contraction of the overloaded right ventricle. Pulmonary diastolic murmurs are uncommon before surgery, but pulmonary incompetence not infrequently follows valvotomy. In pulmonary artery stenosis, the auscultatory findings can be confused with those of pulmonary hypertension because pulmonary valve closure is usually loud and often palpable and the second sound is often split.

Patients with Turner's syndrome characterized by 45 rather than 46 chromosomes, amenorrhea, hypertelorism, webbing of the neck, and short stature may have pulmonary stenosis, and a moon-shaped face has also been described in patients with this lesion. Cyanosis is seen only in severe cases. It may be peripheral and due to low cardiac output, or central and due to arterial desaturation as a result of reversed interarterial shunt through a patent foramen ovale. In this case, it is associated with clubbing of the fingers and polycythemia.

Differential Diagnosis

The differential diagnosis of pulmonary stenosis depends on the severity of the lesion and on the anatomic level of the stenosis.

A. Atrial Septal Defect: Mild valvular lesions can resemble or be associated with an atrial septal defect. The systolic murmur and widely split second sound are common to both lesions.

B. Ventricular Septal Defect: Infundibular stenosis may be confused with a small ventricular septal defect because both lesions have a loud, long systolic murmur, best heard to the left of the sternum.

C. Pulmonary Hypertension: Pulmonary artery stenosis tends to be confused with primary pulmonary hypertension or with Eisenmenger's syndrome. The pressure is the main pulmonary artery is raised in these conditions, and the loud second heart sound and evidence of right ventricular overload are common to all of them. Cardiac catheterization is necessary to confirm the diagnosis.

D. Fallot's Tetralogy: When the pulmonary stenosis is moderate or severe and at the valvular or infundibular level, Fallot's tetralogy is the most important differential diagnosis. The ready fall in arterial oxygen saturation with exercise or amyl nitrite inhalation is perhaps the clearest point suggesting a diagnosis of Fallot's tetralogy.

Cardinal Features and Pathogenesis

The cardinal features of Fallot's tetralogy are right ventricular hypertrophy, large ventricular septal defect, right ventricular outflow obstruction, and overriding aorta.

The ventricular septal defect is high in the membranous portion of the septum and large enough to equalize the pressures in the right and left ventricles. The right ventricular obstruction can be either valvular or infundibular or both, and the overriding of the aorta results in ejection of some right ventricular blood directly into the aorta. In some forms of the condition, both great vessels arise from the right ventricle, a condition termed double outlet right ventricle. The principal variable determining the severity of Fallot's tetralogy is the degree of right ventricular outflow obstruction. The site (valvular, infundibular, or both) of obstruction and the degree of overriding of the aorta play little part in determining the size of the pulmonary blood flow (the principal variable is outflow obstruction) because the right and left ventricular pressures are kept equal by the large ventricular defect.

The spectrum of cases of Fallot's tetralogy ranges from cases of pulmonary atresia in which no blood passes through the pulmonary valve to patients with low, moderate, and high pulmonary blood flow. In the mildest cases of pulmonary stenosis, there is even a left-to-right shunt through the ventricular defect and a pulmonary to systemic blood flow of more than 2:1. Physicians disagree about the appropriateness of the term Fallot's tetralogy for patients with mild pulmonary stenosis, who are said to have acyanotic Fallot's tetraolgy. However, the hemodynamic picture in patients with ventricular septal defect large enough to equalize pressures in the 2 ventricles conforms sufficiently to the definition to make the use of the term Fallot's tetralogy acceptable. The most characteristic feature of the condition is the marked drop in arterial oxygen saturation which occurs with exercise. This is not seen in patients with smaller ventricular defects, for these patients, the term ventricular septal defect with pulmonary stenosis is appropriate.

The overall heart size in Fallot's tetralogy varies with the severity of the lesion. In the severest cases, the heart is not enlarged; in fact, it may be smaller than normal. The aorta is usually large and may be right sided. The right ventricle, although hypertrophied, is not large unless there is a left-to-right shunt. There may be poststenotic dilatation of the pulmonary artery if the right ventricular obstruction is at the valve. The left pulmonary artery may be absent in Fallot's tetralogy, but this abnormality, like a right-sided aortic arch, may occur independently.

Clinical Findings

Symptoms and Signs

1. **Cyanosis at birth:** In all but its mildest forms Fallot's tetralogy is detectable at birth when cyanosis (blue baby) is noted. Cyanosis on exercise always occurs, but clubbing of the fingers is not seen in milder cases.
2. **Dyspnea:** Patients with Fallot's tetralogy are always disabled by dyspnea. Some patient say that they are not short of breath, perhaps because they have never experienced normal exercise tolerance, and sometimes it is not until after the lesion has been treated surgically that they realize how short of breath they actually were.
3. **Squatting:** Adopting the squatting position for relief of dyspnea after exercise is almost pathognomonic of Fallot's teratology in children. It is seldom seen in adults, who prefer to relieve dyspnea by sitting down and putting their feet up or by lying down.
4. **Other symptoms:** Chest pain, arrhythmia, and congestive heart failure are rare in Fallot's tetralogy but are more commonly seen in adults than in children. Because the right ventricle never generates a systolic pressure higher than the systemic arterial pressure, the clinical picture is different from that of severe pulmonary stenosis, in which a right ventricular pressure above systemic level can cause chest pain and right heart failure.
5. **Attacks of Faintness:** In some severe cases, especially with infundibular stenosis, the patient is subject to attacks of faintness and cyanosis. The patient seldom presents with these features initially, but they tend to occur later in the course of the disease. The mechanism of these attacks is infundibular muscular spasm, which reduces pulmonary blood flow. The right-to-left shunt increases, and the patient become progressively more hypoxic. Death may occur in the attack, but more commonly, the right ventricular muscle itself becomes hypoxic and dilates, relieving the condition. These attacks rarely persist into adult life and respond to treatment with propranolol or the administration of general anesthetics.

Hemodynamic Findings

The characteristics hemodynamic feature of Fallot's tetralogy is the shunting of blood across the ventricular septal defect dependent on the relative resistance of the systemic and pulmonary circulation. Because the resistance to blood flow to the lung—the pulmonary stenosis is usually fixed, the systemic resistance is of great importance. Systemic vasodilatation due to muscular exercise, arterial hypoxia, fever, pregnancy, and increased environmental temperature tends to increase or produce right-to-left shunting. As a result, the clinical status of patients with Fallot's tetralogy tends to be unstable and varies from day to day with the weather and the patient's activity and environment.

Other Physical and Cardiac Signs

The physical signs of Fallot's tetralogy vary widely according to the severity of the lesion. Growth is retarded in the most severe cases, and cyanosis and clubbing of the fingers and toes are seen in all but the mildest.

a. The pulse is of normal volume because the systemic output is well maintained. The venous pressure is normal, with at most a small a wave visible in the neck.

The heart is quiet, with little right ventricular heave in severe cases. In milder cases, with left-to-right shunts, there is a larger, more hyperdynamic right ventricle. The intensity and length of the murmur arising from right ventricular outflow obstruction vary with the severity of the lesion. In pulmonary atresia or with severe pulmonary stenosis, the pulmonary blood flow may be so small that there is no pulmonary systolic ejection murmur. In such cases, an almost continuous murmur due to collateral bronchial blood flow may be heard, especially over the back. In mild acyanotic cases, the murmur is long and loud. It may be pansystolic and arise from the ventricular septal defect in patients with a left-to-right shunt. Since the outflow obstruction is always severe enough to raise the right ventricular pressure to systemic levels, the pulmonary valve closure sound is usually inaudible. However, it can be detected by phonocardiography.

1. During cyanotic attacks, the pulmonary systolic ejection murmur may become fainter and pulmonary blood flow falls, and relief of the attack may be first detected by hearing an increase in the intensity of the murmur.
2. **Differential Diagnosis**
    a. Fallot's tetralogy must be distinguished from pulmonary stenosis with reversed interatrial shunt. It is not always possible to make the distinction on clinical grounds, and cardiac catheterization is often necessary to make the correct diagnosis. It may sometimes be difficult to distinguish Fallot's tetralogy from Eisenmenger's complex (ventricular septal defect with pulmonary hypertension), especially when Fallot's tetralogy is mild and there is a bidirectional shunt. Adequate cardiac catheterization studies are mandatory before surgery in such cases because exploratory thoracotomy is often fatal in patients with pulmonary hypertension, pulmonary thrombosis. Cerebral embolism or abscess formation is sometimes ween a result of paradoxical embolization from the right heart through the shunt. Infective endocarditis can occur at the site of the ventricular septal defect in mild cases, or on the pulmonary valve, or in both places. It is occasionally seen both before and after palliative surgery. Right heart failure with edema and raised venous pressure is extremely rare, except after surgery.

■ VENTRICULAR SEPTAL DEFECT

Ventricular septal defect without other associated anomalies constitutes about 10% of cases of congenital heart disease seen in adults. The anatomic but clinically irrelevant presence of a ventricular defect is much more common, being found in Fallot's tetralogy. Eisenmenger's complex, and a number of complex congenital lesions. The cardinal features of ventricular septal defect are left-to-right shunt into the right ventricle, increased pulmonary blood flow, and usually a low pulmonary artery pressure. Variable features are the size of the defect (large or small), the site of defect (membranous or muscular), and the presence or absence of associated aortic incompetence. Only a small number of ventricular defects occur in the muscular part of the septum and these may be multiple. The acquired form of the lesion, seen with rupture of a necrotic area in the septum after myocardial infarction, also involves the muscular part of the septum. The size and site of the ventricular defect determines the size of the left-to-right shunt, which in turn determines the clinical picture. Associated aortic incompetence causes further left ventricular enlargement. A left-to-right shunt at the ventricular level produces an increased flow through the left atrium, left ventricle, and right ventricle. The right atrium is the only chamber through which flow is normal.

The clinical spectrum of cases is wide, varying from maladie de Roger, in which a loud murmur and thrill are the only detectable abnormalities, to defects large enough to cause moderate pulmonary hypertension and large left-to-right shunts. Ventricular septal defect is more important in infants and children than in adults. The defect may become smaller or even close spontaneously as the child grows. A significant percentage of the patients seen in infancy with large ventricular septal defects develop pulmonary hypertension or infundibular stenosis, and some die is infancy. This leaves a relatively small number (usually those with milder defects) to grow to adult life pulmonary to systemic flow ratio of 1.5:1 or more, may cause dyspnea after age 10, and large defects with flow ratios of 3:1 or more are rare but are usually associated with dyspnea on exertion. There is usually a history of a heart murmur present since birth.

The physical signs of ventricular septal defect are dominated by the loud pansystolic murmur and thrill, which are present in the third and fourth left intercostals space inside the apex.

In more than half of adult cases, these are the only abnormal physical signs. In patients with large shunts, the pulse in jerky, resembling a miniature water hammer pulse, and the cardiac impulse is hyperdynamic. The increased force of left ventricular contraction, which is associated with ejection of an increased stroke volume out through the aorta and into the low pressure right ventricle, causes a hemodynamic pattern similar to that seen in mitral incompetence.

The increased pulmonary blood flow causes increased flow through the mitral valve, which produces a third heart sound and a short diastolic flow murmur resulting from relative mitral stenosis.

Differential Diagnosis

Ventricular septal defect is readily confused on physical examination with mitral incompetence, infundibular stenosis, ostium primum defects with cleft mitral valves, and hypertrophic obstruction cardiomyopathy. All these lesions can cause a loud pansystolic murmur and thrill in the left chest. Although the differential diagnosis is relatively easy in cases of severe defect, it is more difficult in patients with milder lesions especially those in whom the murmur is the only abnormality. The almost inevitably severe left ventricular hypertrophy seen on the ECG in obstructive cardiomyopathy should distinguish that lesion, but cardiac catheterization is generally indicated to confirm the diagnosis, even though echocardiography, which displays the ventricular septum and the mitral valve so readily, can be most helpful.

Complications

Heart failure, acquired pulmonary hypertension and atrial arrhythmias are all much less common than in atrial septal defect, because so few patients with large ventricular defects are seen in adult life. Systemic hypertension and coronary atherosclerosis may occur in older patients but do not cause the severe problems seen in patients with atrial septal defects, because the size of left-to-right shunt is limited by the size of the defect and is relatively uninfluenced by the compliance of either ventricle.

PATENT DUCTUS ARTERIOSUS

Cardinal Features

Patent ductus arteriosus is the commonest form of aortopulmonary communication. The shunt is from the aorta at a point just distal to the left subclavian artery into the left pulmonary artery. Aortopulmonary window, in which there is a large communication between the proximal aorta and the main pulmonary artery, is a much rarer lesion that is clinically indistinguishable. The size of the aortopulmonary communication determines the size of the left to right shunt, which in turn determines pulmonary arterial pressure, which is usually low.

Patent ductus arteriosus results in an increased flow through the left atrium and left ventricle and also through the aorta and pulmonary artery. Since there is not an increased flow through the right heart, the lesion loads only the left heart.

Patent ductus arteriosus is more than twice as common in females as in males, and the diagnosis is now usually made in infancy or childhood.

Clinical Features

Symptoms and Signs

Symptoms in patients with patent ductus vary with the size of the left-to-right shunt. In hemodynamically insignificant lesions, which constitute more than half of adult cause, the patient is asymptomatic. A murmur has sometimes been present sicne birth, but more commonly the diagnosis is made later in childhood. A false history of rheumatic fever is present in about 10% of cases. The principal symptom is dyspnea on exertion, with palpitation and chest pain much less frequently seen.

The only abnormality in more than half of cases is the typical 'machinery' murmur, heard high in the left chest below the clavicle. It is loudest at the time of the second heart sound. The murmur is not necessarily continuous in infancy and may be mainly systolic up to age 5, perhaps because the pressure difference between the aorta and pulmonary artery is less at this time. In patients with large left-to-right shunts, cardiac enlargement and a prominent hyperdynamic left ventricular impulses are found in patients with the largest shunts, a wide pulse pressure and a collapsing pulse are seen because of the larger left ventricular stroke volume and the rapid runoff of aortic blood into the low pressure pulmonary circulation. Palpable pulmonary valve closure, reversed splitting of the second heart sound, and a diastolic murmur of relative mitral stenosis are found in patients with large shunts. All of these features are seen in aortopulmonary windows; the only distinguishing feature—a murmur heard low down in the third or fourth left interspace is not a reliable indication of the diagnosis.

Differential Diagnosis

Patent ductus arteriosus can only be differentiated from aortopulmonary windows by cardiac catheterization and angiography. The other lesions that have to be distinguished are those causing continuous or near continuous murmurs. A venous hum gives a continuous bruit heard above the clavicle that is abolished by pressing on the veins at the roof of the neck to interfere with blood flow. If is caused by local narrowing of the vein and is often influenced by posture. Aortic valve disease and ventricular septal defect with aortic incompetence cause murmurs that may be continuous but show two peaks, one in mid systole and the other in early diastole. The murmurs of pulmonary artery stenosis and increased collateral bronchial blood flow start late in systole and peak before the second sound. The murmur of coronary arteriovenous fistula is probably the one most readily confused with patent ductus. It is truly continuous, and the fact that it is best heard at the left lower sternal border rather than in the second left interspace may be the only distinguishing feature.

EISENMENGER'S SYNDROME

Cardinal Features and Pathogenesis

The term Eisenmenger's syndrome is used to describe pulmonary hypertension with reversed shunt. By definition, the pulmonary hypertension does not develop in the course of the disease but is seen on initial examination and has been present from birth or early infancy or childhood. The pathogenesis of the pulmonary vascular obstruction is poorly understood. The pulmonary arterial pressure is at or near systemic level and the shunt is either bidirectional or right-to-left.The pulmonary vascular resistance is raised to more than 7.5 mm Hg/L/min and is often in the same range as the systemic vascular resistance. The principal variable is the level at which the shunt takes place. In Eisenmenger's complex, which is the prototype of the lesion, the location is the ventricle, as shown. Because Eisenmenger's original patient had a ventricular defect, the term Eisenmenger's complex is used to indicate the ventricular nature of the defect, as opposed to the more general term Eisenmenger's syndrome, in which the defect may be at any level. The shunt may be at the aortopulmonary, atrioventricular, atrial or ostium primum level, but it is never solely at the level of an ostium secundum atrial defect Complex congenital lesions such as truncus arteriosus, transposition of the great arteries, single atrium or ventricle, or total anomalous venous drainage may be associated with the pulmonary hypertension.

It is thought that the Eisenmenger reaction, which is the development of severe pulmonary vascular disease, may occur in any form of congenital heart disease in which a large pulmonary blood flow or raised left atrial pressure is present in fetal, neonatal, or infant life. Clues to the mechanism of development of this form of pulmonary hypertension must be sought in the neonatal period. In adult patients, the pulmonary vascular disease of Eisenmenger's syndrome is severe enough to rule out closure of the defect or defects.

The right ventricle and pulmonary artery are usually enlarged in Eisenmenger's syndrome. The other chambers that may be enlarged depend on the site of the associated lesion or lesions.

Acquired Pulmonary Hypertension (Eisenmenger Reaction)

Pulmonary hypertension develops after puberty in some patients, usually those with large left-to-right shunts due to ostium secundum atrial septal defects. In these cases, the term 'atrial septal defect with pulmonary hypertension' or 'acquired Eisenmenger syndrome' has been used. In extremely rare cases, pulmonary hypertension develops after puberty in patients with other lesions, e.g. ventricular septal defect or patent ductus arteriosus. Acquired pulmonary hypertension tends to progress more rapidly that the pulmonary vascular lesions seen in the Eisenmenger complex. Acquired pulmonary hypertension is almost entirely restricted to patients with atrial septal defect.

Use of the Term Eisenmenger's Syndrome

Since the clinical features vary little with the site of lesions and the signs of pulmonary hypertension are dominant, it is convenient to group together under the heading Eisenmenger's syndrome. All patients with cardiac defects associated with pulmonary hypertension that has been present since early life. The clinical course of the patient is also independent of the exact anatomic nature of the defect and depends instead on the pulmonary hypertension in practice, the exact anatomic nature of the lesion in adults with Eisenmenger's syndrome remains unproved until autopsy, and associated lesions such as a ventricular defect in addition to a patent ductus arteriosus and an ostium secundum atrial defect can be present without changing the clinical picture.

Eisenmenger's syndrome accounts for about 7% of cases of adult congenital heart disease and is more common in females than in males. In about one-third of cases, ventricular septal defect is the only lesion associated with the pulmonary hypertension.

Clinical Findings

Symptoms and Signs

Patients with Eisenmenger's syndrome are invariably disabled by dyspnea. A murmur or cyanosis is often said to have been present from infancy, and the absence of any history of severe illness in infancy or childhood is striking. Pneumonia, heart failure, feeding problems, and susceptibility to infection, which are common manifestations of large left-to-right shunts in infancy, are not encountered in retrospective reviews of the history of adults with Eisenmenger's syndrome. It appears that pulmonary vascular resistance is raised at or before birth and that the patient has not passed through a phase of high pulmonary blood flow. Whereas dyspnea is invariably present regardless of age, hemoptysis, palpitation chest pain, and fainting attacks may be seen in adolescence and young adult life. Pregnancy is poorly tolerated, and spontaneous abortion is common.

The physical signs are those of pulmonary hypertension. Cyanosis and clubbing of the fingers may be present, and there is often a prominent a wave in the jugular venous pulse. There may be 'differential' cyanosis in patients with a reversed shunt through a patent ductus arteriosus. The shunted blood passes preferentially to the lower part of the body via that ductus and descending aorta. Thus, there may be cyanosis and clubbing of the toes when the hands—especially the right hand is pink and show no clubbing of the fingers. The difference is best seen when the systemic circulation has been subject to vasodilatation, e.g. after a hot shower or bath. These clinical findings can be confirmed by finding a difference in the oxygen content (or saturation) between right brachial and femoral blood samples.

The heart is usually not much enlarged and is often quiet. A right ventricular heave may be present, and pulmonary valve closure is often palpable. There is usually a systolic ejection click, followed by a short systolic ejection murmur over the pulmonary artery and a loud single second heart sound. As early diastolic murmur of pulmonary incompetence is common, and the clearest examples of this murmur (Graham Steell murmur) are encountered in Eisenmenger's syndrome. Signs of congestive heart failure are seldom seen, but progressive cyanosis and polycythemia are common.

Differential Diagnosis

Eisenmenger's syndrome must be distinguished from pulmonary hypertension due to acquired lesions that raise left atrial pressure. Tight mitral stenosis is by far the commonest of these lesions, but rare lesions such as left atrial myxoma, cor triatriatum, and sclerosing mediastinitis with pulmonary venous obstruction may occur. Primary (idiopathic) and thromboembolic pulmonary hypertension should also be excluded because such conditions carry a worse prognosis than Eisenmenger's syndrome. The history of a murmur and cyanosis dating back to infancy is of great help in identifying congenital lesions but is not always available. In some patients with severe acquired pulmonary hypertension, opening of the foramen ovale may cause right-to-left shunting and lead to an erroneous diagnosis of a congenital lesion. Complete cardiac catheterization studies may be needed, including measurements of the effects of oxygen and vasodilator drugs on pulmonary vascular resistance. Pulmonary artery stenosis may also be a possible cause of the physical signs of increased pressure in the main pulmonary artery.

◼ COARCTATION OF THE AORTA

Cardinal Features and Pathogenesis

This obstructive aortic lesion, which is characteristically associated with hypertension in the upper half of the body, with lower pressure in the legs, is usually diagnosed in childhood. The obstruction almost invariably is in the aortic isthmus just distal to the origin of the left subclavian artery and at the level where the ductus arteriosus joins the descending aorta. The obstruction may rarely be at over sites in the aorta. There is usually poststenotic dilatation of the aorta distal to the site of obstruction. Collateral vessels develop that tend to bypass the obstruction. The principal variable in the lesion is the severity of the obstruction, which varies from complete aortic atresia to slight narrowing, and the size of the collateral vessels. These can be so large that a minimal pressure difference is present between the ascending and descending aorta in a patient with complete aortic obstruction at the site of coarctation.

In coarctation of the aorta, the left ventricle is hypertrophied and enlarged in proportion to the severity of the lesion. The proximal aorta is distended, and there is poststenotic dilatation of the aorta distal to the obstruction.

Coarctation of the aorta is associated with a number of other left sided congenital lesions, namely bicuspid aortic valve, patent ductus arteriosus, aortic stenosis, ventricular septal defect, mitral stenosis, aortic or mitral atresia, and other hypoplastic left heart syndromes. One theory of the cause of coarctation is that the specialized tissue in the ductus arteriosus near the area of the isthmus of the aorta (which constricts with the rise in aortic oxygen tension at birth) spills over into the aorta and causes constriction at this site in addition to or instead of narrowing at the ductus. Coarctation of the aorta represents about 5% of cases of adult congenital heart disease and is more common in males than in females by a factor of more than 3:1. Some clinically insignificant narrowing of the aorta at the isthmus of the aorta is common, even in the absence of hypertension. This should not be emphasized, however, and the use of the term pseudocoarctation to describe such a condition is not endorsed.

Clinical Findings

Symptoms and Signs

Coarctation of the aorta produces few symptoms. The lesion is usually discovered by finding an abnormally high blood pressure or a systolic murmur. Dyspnea on exertion, headache, and throbbing in the head are sometimes seen. In older, untreated cases, intermittent claudication may occur. Left heart failure, with pulmonary congestion and edema, occurs late in the disease, even in cases presenting in adult life.

a. The diagnosis of coarctation of the aorta can be readily made on physical examination. The carotid arteries shows well marked, bounding pulsations resulting from the forceful ejection of the left ventricular stroke volume into the reduced capacity of the arterial bed. There is usually a prominent pulsation in the suprasternal notch. The level of arterial pressure varies considerably with the age of the patient, being higher in older persons. The pulse pressure in the arms is wide, whereas that in the leg is reduced. The femoral pulses may be absent in severe cases; if they are present, the characteristic sign of delay between the timing of the upstrokes of the radial and femoral pulses should be sought. The examiner should time locate the femoral pulse with one hand and then palpate the radial pulse to detect and time the difference between the arrival of the two waves. The pulses are synchronous in normal subjects, whereas delays of 0.1 sec are readily discernible in patients with coarctation. Collateral vessels are often present on the back. They are best seen and felt by feeling the intercostals arteries under the ribs and the enlarged arteries around the scapula as the patient bends forward.

Cardiac Signs

The heart is often enlarged, with a prominent left ventricular heave. Two varieties of murmur in coarctation of the aorta can usually be distinguished. One arises from the aortic obstruction and is late systolic in timing and ejection in type. The other is longer and more continuous and arises from the collateral vessels. Both are heard best in the back. The aortic valve closure sound is loud, and a third heart sound and a short delayed diastolic murmur arising from the mitral valve are occasionally heard.

Estein's malformation is a rare congenital malformation that represents about 1% of cases of adult congenital heart disease. It presents a sufficiently characteristic clinical picture to warrant separate description.

The basic abnormality is downward displacement of the tricuspid valve, with atrialization of a large part of the right ventricle. The principal variable is the presence or absence of an associated ostium secundum atrial defect. The atrialized portion of the ventricle hinders rather than helps the forward flow of blood, and the tricuspid valve is congenitally incompetent. The lesion is remakably well tolerated and was first recognized clinically in a cyanotic form in patients who also had an atrial septal defect. More acyanotic cases without atrial defects have come to be recognized, and it now appears that the lesion probably occurs more commonly without an atrial defect. Pulmonary blood flow is reduced, especially when right-to-left shunting through an atrial defect is present.

CLINICAL FINDINGS
Symptoms and Signs

Dyspnea and fatigue are the commonest presenting symptoms. Atrial arrhythmias commonly cause palpitations, and right heart failure occurs with increasing age. The pulse is of small amplitude, and the venous pressure is usually riased in adult patients. Atrial fibrillation is usually present after age 20. The heart is quiet, with distant heart sounds. There is usually a systolic murmur of tricuspid origin and wide splitting of the second heart sound. A short scratchy diastolic murmur or third heart sound arising from the tricuspid valve is usually heard at the left sternal edge. The murmurs tend to increase in intensity during inspiration.

DIFFERENTIAL DIAGNOSIS

Massive cardiac enlargement due to pericardial disease can usually be distinguished on the basis of the history. The cardiac enlargement will have developed recently, whereas in Ebstein's malformation there is a long history of heart disease. Severe right heart failure in patients with congenital pulmonary stenosis may produce a somewhat similar picture, and advanced rheumatic tricuspid valve disease can be recognized and ruled out because there will almost certainly be some associated mitral valve disease.

Tricuspid Atresia

In cases of atresia of the tricuspid valve, there must be an atrial defect through which all the systemic venous return reaches the left heart. As a result, there is left ventricular hypertrophy that shows up clearly on the ECG as left ventricular dominance because the right ventricle is absent or not functional. Various associated lesions, especially transposition of great arteries, may be present, and the origin of blood flow to the lungs is the principal variable. There may be associated pulmonary atresia with reduced pulmonary blood flow, or there may be a ventricular septal defect through which an increased pulmonary blood flow reaches the lungs. In rare cases, the tricuspid atresia is not complete, and there is a small under-developed right ventricle. In such patients, the characteristic finding of the lesion (left ventricular hypertrophy on the ECG) is still present. A right ventricular prosthesis interposed between the right atrium and the pulmonary artery (if one exists) is now the treatment of choice. Previously, an anastomosis was made between the superior vena cava and the right pulmonary artery (Glenn's operation). This is a condition in which cyanosis is associated with LVH not RVH.

Total Anomalous Pulmonary Venous Drainage

In this lesion, all the blood returning from the lungs enters the right heart. There must be necessity of an atrial septal defect. The principal variable is the route taken by the pulmonary venous return, which is most commonly via a left-sided superior vena cava to the in-nominate vein and thence to the right atrium via the superior vena cava. The other common pattern seen in infancy is via the inferior vena cava below the diaphragm. More rarely, other patterns of venous return are seen. The pulmonary blood flow and blood pressure vary, and the pulmonary venous return may be obstructed, leading to pulmonary venous congestion and edema. The variety of the lesion most commonly seen in older children is the pattern involving the in-nominate vein. The venous return is free, and there is usually raised pulmonary vascular resistance. In this lesion, there is a characteristic chest X-ray picture called "snowman heart". The upper circular shadow is the anomalous venous pathway, which lies above the lower circular shadow formed by the rest of the heart.

Other Lesions

Always palpate for apex beat if not found on left and heart sounds better on right side. Dextrocardia with a mirror image heart in the right side of the chest can occur, with or without any other lesion, although situs inversus of the abdominal viscera is usually present. Dextroversion of the heart with abnormal rotation that leaves the heart mainly in the right chest can also occur. In this case, the cardiac chambers are not in a mirror image position. Complete atrioventricular block may be occur as an isolated congenital lesion or in association with other congenital heart lesions. Complete atrioventricular block is also a non-infrequent complication of cardiac surgery performed to relieve congenital heart lesions.

Chapter 4

Valvular Heart Disease

Both undergraduate and postgraduate students invariably get cases of valvular heart disease (Rheumatic mostly but sometimes nonrheumatic also) Valvular heart disease presents some of the most important diagnostic problems in adult cardiology. Because of the vast range in types of lesions, valvular involvement, causes, and associated conditions, certain broad generalizations about valvular heart disease are inevitable.

CLASSIFICATION OF VALVULAR DISEASE

Valvular disease can be classified according to the following factors :

A. **Lesions:** Valvular disease can be divided into three categories on the basis of the type of lesion: stenosis, incompetence, and mixed stenosis and incompetence (regurgitation, insufficiency).

B. **Valvular Involvement:** Lesions involving the mitral and aortic valves are more common than tricuspid and pulmonary valve lesions in adult valvular disease.

C. **Causes:** Rheumatic endocarditis is the most important cause of valvular heart disease; degenerative disorders and congenital disease are other prominent causes.

Associated lesions such as past or present myocardial damage due to rheumatic carditis, or degenerative changes due to hypertension, atherosclerosis. Cardiomyopathy or abnormal wear and tear secondary to the valvular lesion will affect the classification.

Variation in clinical features: Because the course of chronic valvular disease often lasts for 20–30 years, it is much easier to gain experience based on several patients seen at different stages of the disease that it is to follow a single patient progressively through the different stages. Although it is relatively easy to see that disease has progressed in a given patient, the nature, timing, and rate of progress are difficult to determine. The natural progress of disease is also modified by treatment, and it is in valvular heart disease that the iatrogenic modification of cardiac disease is seen most clearly.

Acute Valvular Lesions: The clinical picture in patients with acute valvular lesions is different from that seen in classic chronic lesions associated with rheumatic fever. Pure valvular incompetence rather than stenosis is an example of the classic acute lesion. It has become increasingly important to distinguish the clinical features of an acute lesion, which develops over a period of minutes, days, or weeks-from the more readily recognized effects of chronic valvular lesions. Acute lesions are relatively rate (10%), and their importance depends on their severity. If the patient survives, the onset of an acute lesion, compensatory responses to increased cardiac load occur, leading to hypertrophy or dilatation of the appropriate chambers. Such a lesion becomes chronic in about 1 year. In acute severe valvular lesions, the heart tolerates the extra load poorly. In acute aortic and mitral incompetence, pulmonary congestion and edema tend to so dominate the clinical picture that separate clinical features must be distinguished. The lungs carry the brunt of the disease, and some of the cardiac manifestations associated with chronic valvular lesions may not appear for several weeks.

MITRAL VALVE DISEASE

Mitral valve disease is the commonest from of valvular heart disease and accounts for more than half of cases with significant valvular lesions. Rheumatic heart disease is the commonest cause of mitral valve disease in particular and all valve disease in general. Acute clinical manifestations of rheumatic fever are detected in only about half of patients who subsequently develop mitral valve disease. The presence or absence of a history or rheumatic fever makes no difference in the course of the disease or in its clinical, hemodynamic, or pathologic finding. In patients who have no history of rheumatic fever, it is generally assumed that a subclinical attack without over signs of cardiac or joints involvement was responsible for the valvular lesion.

Classification of Mitral Valve Disease

Mitral valve disease has been classified somewhat arbitrarily into three types: mitral stenosis, mixed mitral stenosis and incompetence, and mitral incompetence.

It is difficult to distinguish between the different lesions in some cases, and in some patients, the disease can on occasion shift from one category to another. The classification depends primarily on the physical finding rather than the history, although the history and course of the disease vary in the different lesions.

In mitral stenosis, the predominant lesion is obstruction to the diastolic flow of blood through the mitral valve. The hallmark of the lesion is the presence of a presystolic (atrial systolic) murmur indicating that mitral flow is still continuing when atrial contraction occurs and that the patient is still in sinus rhythm. Atrial fibrillation commonly accompanies mitral valve disease and occurs in all types of lesions. In mitral stenosis, however, it is seldom present when the patient first presents with symptoms. Predominant obstruction to mitral valve flow during diastole is such a potent cause of symptoms that patients with this lesion develop dyspnea early is adult life in all but the mildest cases.

In *mixed mitral stenosis and incompetence*, there is both obstruction to forward flow and leakage of blood from the left ventricle into the left atrium during systole. Mitral stenosis and incompetence have traditionally been thought to be mutually exclusive lesions that cannot coexist except in a mild form. The rationale for this category of mixed stenosis and incompetence may alter the natural history of mitral valve disease. In relieving mitral stenosis, the surgeon non-infrequently renders the valve incompetent. Long-term follow-up of patients who have had mitral valvotomy shows that the operation is usually only palliative and that symptoms recur. Although some patients show evidence of restenosis, the majority present a clinical picture of mixed stenosis and incompetence, often with a fixed, calcified valve that neither opens nor shuts completely. The hallmark of the lesion is the absence of a presystolic murmur, which indicates that the obstruction is not severe enough to hinder forward flow at the end of diastole. It also implies that the patient is in atrial fibrillation. Patients with mixed mitral stenosis and incompetence characteristically develop symptoms for the first time when their cardiac rhythm changes sinus to atrial fibrillation. This usually takes place at about age 40. This course also occurs in some patients who have not had a previous mitral valvotomy.

Mitral incompetence differs from other kind of mitral valve disease in that it has several forms and has a variety of causes. It is here divided into the following categories: (1) acute mitral incompetence and (2) chronic mitral incompetence (hemodynamically insignificant and significant). The hallmark of mitral incompetence is the presence of a systolic murmur without any significant diastolic murmur to indicate the presence of obstruction to the diastolic forward flow across the valve. In acute lesions the onset is abrupt and caused by acute disruption of the mitral valve due to rupture or stretching of the chordae tendineae, weakening of the papillary muscles, or perforation of a valve cusp. In hemodynamically insignificant chromic lesions, the characteristic feature is a late systolic murmur with or without a midsystolic ejection click. The murmur is associated with a specific clinical picture (click-murmur syndrome) and a course that may lead in time to either a significant chronic lesion or an acute exacerbation. In chromic hemodynamically significant chronic lesions the characteristic feature is a late systolic murmur with or without a midystolic ejection click. The murmur is associated with a specific clinical picture (click-murmur syndrome) and a course that may lead in time to either a significant chronic lesion or an acute exacerbation. In chronic hemodynamically significant mitral incompetence there is a pansystolic murmur with a third heart sound and no diastolic murmur. The lesion is well tolerated, and even the onset of atrial fibrillation does not cause serious symptoms. Left ventricular stroke volume is increased in mitral incompetence, and the way the ventricle responds to the extra "flow" work determines the course of the disease.

Cause of Mitral Valve Disease

Rheumatic heart disease is, in effect, the sole cause of all mitral valve disease except mitral incompetence. Even in cases of mitral incompetence, however, rheumatic fever probably accounts for half of chronic lesions. Rheumatic heart disease is much more common in women than in men; the female: male ratio of 9:1 in mitral stenosis falls to 3:1 in mixed mitral

stenosis and incompetence and 1:1 in mitral stenosis or mixed stenosis and incompetence are congenital heart disease and hypertrophic cardiomyopathy. Congenital heart disease is rare, being encountered in less than 1% of adult cases, and it is debatable whether hypertrophic cardiomyopathy should be considered as a form of mitral disease or as part of the differential diagnosis.

MITRAL STENOSIS

In mitral stenosis, rheumatic endocarditis scars the mitral valve and commonly causes fusion of the commissures and matting of the chordae tendineae, which interfere with the opening of the valve. The left atrium bears the brunt of the load, and the extent to which it dilates depends on its internal pressure and the state of the atrial myocardium. With time, calcification of the mitral valve renders it less mobile. In some patients with tight mitral stenosis, pulmonary vascular resistance rises because the pulmonary arteriolar venous pressure by vasoconstriction. The reasons for this response are not clear. The increase in resistance appears to be related to the rise in pulmonary venous pressure and does not occur when the rise is small. At first, the changes are functional and reversible by drugs such as acetylcholine and tolazoline. Later, however, anatomic changes appear, with medial hypertrophy and intimal thickening of pulmonary arterioles occurring first at the base of the lungs, where venous pressure is higher because of the effects of gravity, and later throughout the lungs. Severe pulmonary vascular lesions with markedly raised pulmonary vascular resistance (> 7.5 mm Hg/L/min) are virtually limited to patients with severe mitral stenosis, whereas lesser increases in pulmonary vascular resistance are seen in other forms of mitral disease. When pulmonary vascular resistance rises, the course of mitral stenosis is strikingly altered; the brunt of the load is transferred from the left ventricle, and right ventricular failure eventually occurs if the stenosis is not relieved.

Passive pulmonary hypertension: The pulmonary arterial pressure must rise to maintain pulmonary blood flow in any patient whose left artrial pressure rises. Thus, when left atrial pressure rises to 25–30 mm Hg in mitral stenosis, the pulmonary arterial mean pressure inevitably increases to a mean level of 30–40 mm Hg. This "passive" pulmonary hypertension results in redistribution of the blood flow to the lungs, with more perfusion of the apexes. The load is not severe enough to cause right heart failure and pulmonary congestion with orthopnea and paroxysmal dyspnea dominates the clinical picture. Before mitral valvotomy was available, some patients died of acute pulmonary edema. The right ventricle continued to pump blood into the congested lung, the leakage of fluid into the alveoli flooded the lungs, and produced a fatal disturbance of gas exchange.

Onset of Atrial Fibrillation

In patients without pulmonary hypertension, atrial fibrillation usually develops with the passage of time. Even if pulmonary hypertension is present, 30% of patients develop atrial fibrillation early in the course of the disease. Atrial fibrillation is most closely correlated with age, but it also depends on left atrial pressure and the severity of involvement of the left atrium in the rheumatic process.

Clinical Findings

Symptoms

1. **Dyspnea:** The commonest presenting symptom (80%) in patients with mitral stenosis is shortness of breath on exertion. In women with severe lesions, this is usually noticed in early adult life (age 20–30 years), while the patient is still in sinus rhythm, perhaps during pregnancy. The dyspnea is due to pulmonary congestion that results from a rise in left atrial pressure associated with an increase in heart rate and a decrease in left atrial emptying time. The increased stiffness of the lungs increases the work of breathing, and the fall in cardiac output, which results from mitral value obstruction leads to an increase in heart rate the further aggravates the congestion. Any factor that increases the, heart rate is likely to aggravate dyspnea in mitral stenosis; anxiety, anemia, exposure to high altitude, pregnancy, thyrotoxicosis, and atrial fibrillation in a patient, with significant mitral stenosis virtually always provokes dyspnea. In milder cases, there may have been no dyspnea prior to the onset of arrhythmia, but in most instances the onset of atrial fibrillation exacerbates dyspnea rather than provoking it for the first time. Conversely, when a patient believed to have significant mitral stenosis develops atrial fibrillation without experiencing dyspnea, the diagnosis is in doubt and the lesion is at most mild.

2. **Paroxysmal nocturnal dyspnea**: The dyspnea in patients with mitral stenosis may be severe enough to progress to episodes of acute pulmonary edema, especially in the presence of some additional stress. Increased heart rate due to anxiety, atrial arrhythmia, fever due to intercurrent infection, excessive salt intake, or unaccustomed exertion should be sought. An acute episode of dyspnea often occurs at night, and the patient wakes from sleep with a choking sensation accompanied by cough. Relief is obtained by sitting or standing up. One episode of paroxysmal nocturnal dyspnea may cause the patient to sleep on several pillows indefinitely, and the association between recumbency and dyspnea is readily apparent to the patient. However, orthopnea is not necessarily present just because the patient uses several pillows. It is important to count the pulse and respirations and observe how well a change in posture is tolerated when the patient lies flat. Orthopnea should be treated as a sign rather than a symptom.

3. **Hemoptysis**: Hemoptysis is the second most common presenting symptom in mitral

stenosis. There may be frank pulmonary hemorrhage from rupture of a pulmonary vein; frothy pink, blood-tinged sputum in pulmonary edema; or hemoptysis resulting from pulmonary infarction. Hemoptysis is seen in patients with raised pulmonary vascular resistance and in those with pulmonary congestion.

4. **Systemic embolism**: Presenting symptoms due to systemic embolism are infrequent in patients with mitral stenosis. Embolism is more common after atrial fibrillation has occurred and tends to occur later in the disease.

5. **Palpitations**: Palpitations are rarely the chief presenting complaint. Any arrhythmia is likely to provoke dyspnea, and the patient will usually complain of dyspnea rather than palpitations.

6. **Symptoms in patients with raised pulmonary vascular resistance**: Fatigue, coldness of the extremities, abdominal discomfort, and swelling of the abdomen and ankles are symptoms of right heart involvement. They suggest the presence of severe pulmonary hypertension and raised pulmonary vascular resistance with a low cardiac output and are thus indicative of severe mitral stenosis. Symptoms of right heart involvement can also occur in patients with associated organic involvement of the tricuspid valve. Chest pain that is indistinguishable from angina pectoris is occasionally noted in the presence of raised pulmonary vascular resistance or pulmonary embolism.

7. **Episodic symptoms**: Confusion in diagnosis sometimes occurs when the patient's symptoms are episodic. In this case, arrhythmia should be suspected, and the physician should try to see the patient during an attack in order to record an ECG.

Signs

The physical signs in patients with mitral stenosis vary with the severity of the valvular lesion and also with the amount of increase in pulmonary vascular resistance. The classic signs of mitral stenosis develop early in the natural course of the condition and can usually be noted before symptoms develop. However, the patient may have to engage in exercise in order to elicit the signs. In classic mitral stenosis, the pulse is normal or small in amplitude, and the blood pressure and systemic venous pressure are normal.

1. **Loud first heart sound**: The heart is not enlarged, and on palpation, there is an obvious localized tapping cardiac impulse. This represents the vibrations from the loud first heart sound that result from closure of the mitral valve (closing snap). There may also be a diastolic thrill with presystolic accentuation felt at the apex and a palpable opening snap felt at the base of the heart.

2. **Opening snap**: On auscultation, the first sound is loud, and the second sound is followed by a loud opening snap that is high-pitched and widely transmitted but heard best to the left of the sternum, near the base of the heart.

3. **Diastolic murmur with presystolic accentuation**: The characteristic finding in predominant mitral stenosis is a long, loud, rumbling mitral diastolic murmur with presystolic accentuation due to atrial systole. The murmur is often best heard in a localized area about 2.5 cm in diameter located at the apex of the heart. The patient should lie on the left side after exercise, and the physician should use the bell of the stethoscope and little pressure on the chest. The murmur may be absent in mid-diastole in mild cases but still show presystolic accentuation.

4. **S_2-OS interval**: The time elapsing between the aortic valve closure sound and the opening snap is roughly related to left atrial pressure. If left atrial pressure is high, the valve will open early because left atrial pressure soon comes to exceed left ventricular pressure. Conversely, if left atrial pressure is low, a longer time will elapse before left atrial

pressure exceeds left ventricular pressure and filling starts. Thus, an early opening snap (0.05–0.07 sec after A2) suggests more severe stenosis than a later (0.10–0.12 sec after A2) opening snap. The presence of loud opening and closing snaps indicates that the mitral valve is flexible and suggests that mitral valvotomy rather than valve replacement will be appropriate treatment.

There is not infrequently a mitral systolic murmur in pure mitral stenosis. A long, rumbling diastolic murmur with presystolic accentuation during atrial contraction is the definitive auscultatory sign of mitral stenosis, and the presence of a presystolic (atrial systolic) murmur excludes a diagnosis of significant mitral incompetence. Thus, even though mild, hemodynamically insignificant mitral incompetence may cause a systolic murmur, this should not be construed as evidence of significant mitral incompetence when a patient has none of the other signs of mitral incompetence but some of the signs of mitral stenosis. The murmur may be due to tricuspid incompetence.

5. **Signs in the presence of atrial fibrillation**: When the patient develops atrial fibrillation, the presystolic murmur disappear. The heart rate becomes irregular, and after the heart rate has been slowed by digitalis therapy, it becomes important to listen for the length of the diastolic murmur during the longest diastolic pauses. In patients with predominant mitral stenosis, the murmur should persist until the end of diastole even in cardiac cycles lasting 1 sec. A shorter murmur suggests either mixed mitral stenosis and incompetence or raised pulmonary vascular resistance. It is the length of the diastolic murmur and not the fact that it lasts until the next first heart sound that is important in the determination of the severity of mitral stenosis.

6. **Pulmonary signs**: Rales at the bases of the lungs are commonly found in mitral stenosis, but their absence does not exclude the possibility of pulmonary congestion or even edema. The patient is often orthopneic because the lungs become more congested when the patient is in a supine position, the respiratory rate increase as the lungs become stiffer, and the patient becomes breathless. It is more reliable to have the patient lie flat and look for evidence of orthopnea than to ask shortness of breath occurs on recumbency.

7. **Signs in the presence of pulmonary hypertension**: When pulmonary vascular resistance is markedly raised (> 7.5 mm Hg/L/min), the physical signs of mitral stenosis tend to be different. The patient usually has a low cardiac output and is often thin, with peripheral cyanosis, cool extremities, and a pulse of small volume. Dilated veins on the cheeks combined with peripheral cyanosis give rise to a "mitral facies" that is also seen in other patients with a chronically low cardiac output. Systemic venous pressure is likely to be raised, with a prominent a wave visible in the jugular pulse if sinus rhythm is present. The heart may be enlarged, with a right ventricular substernal impulse. The auscultatory signs of mitral stenosis tend to be less florid than those in patients with low pulmonary vascular resistance because the cardiac output is lower. Less often, there is a diastolic thrill, but pulmonary valve closure is usually palpable. In about one-third of cases, either reduction in the cardiac output or valvular calcification modifies the classic physical signs, making the diagnosis difficult. Calcification of the valve may eliminate the opening snap but should not affect the murmur. Low output may eliminate the murmur but should not affect the snap. Calcification of the mitral valve does not always affect the physical signs and more than half of patients with valvular calcification have an opening snap. There is often a pulmonary systolic ejection click and a short pulmonary systolic murmur in addition to a loud pulmonary valve closure sound.

a. **Pulmonary incompetence**: Pulmonary incompetence secondary to pulmonary hypertension may cause an immediate diastolic murmur at the base of the heart (Graham Steel murmur). In practice, associated hemodynamically insignificant aortic incompetence is a much more common cause of such a basal murmur.

b. **Tricuspid incompetence**: Pansystolic murmurs are common in patients with pulmonary hypertension and are usually due to secondary tricuspid incompetence, as shown by increased systemic venous pressure, a prominent a wave in the neck, and increased intensity of the murmur during inspiration. When right ventricular failure occurs, the right side of the heart may become so large that it occupies the whole front of the chest.

8. **Signs in the presence of low output:** In severely ill patients, the mitral diastolic murmur may vary in intensity because of changes in cardiac output or heart rate. The face that one observer has heard the murmur and another has not, should not be discounted, and repeated examinations may be helpful. A mitral diastolic murmur that is ordinarily inaudible may be heard by listening in the axilla, with the patient lying on the left side.

9. **Assessment of severity from physical signs:** Assessment of the severity of mitral stenosis based on physical signs is not of sufficient accuracy to be clinically valid. Patients with varying degrees of stenosis can all show fully developed classic physical signs. The timing of the opening snap confirmed by phonocardiography may be a guide to the severity of the disease, but this measurement must be assessed in relation to the rest of the clinical picture. The degree of pulmonary congestion shown on the chest X-ray and the findings at cardiac catheterization provide a more reliable index of severity.

Differential Diagnosis

Left atrial myxoma is the most important disorder in the differential diagnosis of mitral stenosis with or without raised pulmonary vascular resistance. The radiologic picture closely resembles that of mitral stenosis, and left atrial appendage enlargement is seen. Episodic symptoms, variable heart murmurs, fever, systemic embolism, a raised sedimentation rate, and hyperglobulinemia suggest the possibility of myxoma. The lesion is 100 times less common than mitral stenosis and 100 times more common than the rare congenital lesion cor triatriatum, in which the left atrium is divided into an upper and a lower chamber by an incomplete transverse septum. Cor triatriatum may also simulate stenosis. Echocardiography and angiocardiography with injection of dye into the left ventricle or pulmonary artery are helpful in diagnosis.

In patients with raised pulmonary vascular resistance, pulmonary hypertension due to any other cause such as Eisenmenger's syndrome, idiopathic or thromboembolic pulmonary hypertension, or atrial septal defect with acquired pulmonary hypertension must be ruled out. Because mitral stenosis with pulmonary hypertension can be cured by surgery and patients with pulmonary hypertension due to other causes do not withstand exploratory thoracotomy well, it is essential to make the correct diagnosis.

A. **Atrial Fibrillation**: Atrial fibrillation occurs so frequently in the course of mitral stenosis that it hardly qualifies as a complication. The importance of both the effect of atrial fibrillation on the natural history of the lesion and its time of onset cannot be stressed too strongly. The circumstances precipitating atrial fibrillation and its clinical effects provide important diagnostic and prognostic information about the lesion. It is important to determine whether the onset of atrial fibrillation aggravated existing symptoms or heralded their appearance. If the onset of atrial fibrillation escapes notice in a patient with mitral stenosis, either the lesion is extremely mild or increased pulmonary vascular resistance is present. In the latter situation, the patient has presumably been so disabled that the additional stress of the arrhythmia goes unnoticed. The earlier atrial fibrillation occurs, the worse the prognosis because of the implication that rheumatic carditis must have damaged the atrial muscle. Conversely, if atrial fibrillation has not developed by age 50 in a patient with mitral stenosis, the stenosis is almost invariably mild. It is therefore imperative to determine the circumstance surrounding the onset of atrial fibrillation and to assess the patient's tolerance of the arrhythmia.

B. **Bronchitis:** The congested lungs of patients with mitral disease are prone to bronchitis. This is seen more frequently in patients with mitral stenosis because pulmonary congestion is generally more severe than in other type of mitral valve disease.

C. **Pulmonary Infarction**: Pulmonary embolism and pulmonary infarction are common, especially in mitral stenosis with raised pulmonary vascular resistance. The lungs with their double arterial blood supply normally are not subject to infarction unless they are congested, and mitral stenosis is one of the commonest conditions in which pulmonary embolism is followed by pulmonary infarction. It is not always possible to determine the origin of the thrombus, and although emboli from the veins of the pelvis and legs are common, the possibility of thrombosis in situ should not be ruled out.

MIXED MITRAL STENOSIS AND INCOMPETENCE

In some cases, the rheumatic involvement of the mitral valve leads to dilatation and stretching of the valve tissue and subsequent scarring and retraction in addition to narrowing. In this case, stenosis is present in addition to significant leakage through the valve. After severe mitral stenosis has been treated surgically, the stenosis is less severe, but the valve is still abnormal. With time, degenerative changes, fibrosis and calcification stiffen and immobilize the valve and produce a mixture of stenosis and incompetence. The cardinal features of this lesion include obstruction and leakage at the mitral valve, left atrial enlargement, and left ventricular enlargement (not hypertrophy). Variable features, which may alter these findings, are the severity of obstruction, the amount of regurgitation, and the severity of rheumatic myocardial damage.

Patients with mixed mitral stenosis and incompetence run a more constant clinical course than might be expected in view of the numerous possible combinations of severity of the components. The blood that leaks back across the mitral valve during systole must flow forward during diastole, augmenting the normal forward stroke volume. Mitral incompetence thus increases mitral diastolic blood flow. The extra blood flow resulting from systolic mitral incompetence raises left atrial pressure and makes any mitral stenosis appear more severe. For these reasons, the clinical severity of mixed mitral stenosis and incompetence depends on the sum of the incompetence and the stenosis and tends to remain constant. If there is more stenosis than incompetence, there is a smaller amount of systolic back flow and a smaller diastolic forward flow across the valve. If there is more incompetence than stenosis, there is a larger systolic backflow and a larger diastolic forward flow. Thus, the symptoms in patients with mixed mitral lesions tend to vary less than might be expected. In contrast, the physical signs—which depend mainly on the volume of blood passing through the mitral valve during both systole and diastole—tend to depend on the severity of incompetence, and there is wide variation in the lengths and intensities of the systolic and diastolic mitral murmurs and in the degree of left ventricular volume overload.

Clinical Findings

Symptoms

1. **Dyspnea:** Dyspnea is the commonest presenting symptom in patients with mixed mitral stenosis and incompetence. It seldom occurs while the patients are in sinus rhythm. The patient often presents with an acute episode of dyspnea associated with the development of atrial fibrillation. This onset commonly heralds the approach of other symptoms, and the patient, who may have been living a relatively normal life, becomes acutely ill with severe dyspnea and perhaps pulmonary edema. Atrial fibrillation is sometimes triggered by an intercurrent infection such as influenza, pneumonia and a systemic or pulmonary embolism may occur simultaneously. This clinical picture is so common that it is important to consider the possibility of mitral stenosis and incompetence in any patient who suddenly becomes short of breath, especially if the heart rate is rapid and atrial fibrillation is present. The physical signs can be difficult to interpret in the acute stage when the heart rate is rapid. Episodic dyspnea may be present when there is paroxysmal atrial arrhythmia. In such circumstances, it is important to see the patient during an attack.

2. **Palpitations**: Palpitations are common in patients with mixed mitral stenosis and incompetence. Palpitations are generally due to atrial arrhythmia; if the heart rate is rapid, dyspnea is likely to occur.

3. **Systemic embolism:** The first symptom of mixed mitral stenosis and incompetence may be due to acute systemic embolism. Sudden pain and coldness in the leg, sudden paralysis, acute loin pain due to renal infarction, flank pain due to infarction of the spleen, and infarction of the bowel due to mesenteric artery emboli sometimes occur. Embolism usually occurs in patients with atrial fibrillation, particularly when the rhythm changes, but it may happen when the patient is in sinus rhythm.

4. **Pressure from a large left atrium:** Symptoms due to pressure from a greatly enlarged left atrium on surrounding structures are occasionally seen. Thus, cough, hoarseness, and recurrent lung infection involving the left lower lobe may occur.

Signs

The signs in patients with mixed mitral, stenosis and incompetence. When incompetence is the predominant lesion, the left ventricular systolic ejection rate is more rapid than normal, and the peripheral pulse resembles a miniature "water-hammer" pulse. In patients with mixed mitral stenosis and incompetence, it is not always easy to assess the relative importance of the stenosis, the incompetence, or the overall severity of the lesion. It is possible that the patients with this lesion have resulted from either valvotomy or calcification and fixation of the deformed valve as well as degenerative, age-related changes and increased wear and tear.

The systemic venous pressure is not often raised unless there is associated tricuspid valve disease. Because pulmonary hypertension is seldom severe, the pulse is usually normal and the rhythm irregular in patients with atrial fibrillation. The heart is usually enlarged, with a hyperdynamic left ventricular impulse. The first sound may be loud and there may be an opening snap, especially if the patient has had a previous valvotomy for mitral stenosis. A third heart sound may also be heard, sometimes replacing the snap rather than accompanying it. Depending on the volume of mitral diastolic blood flow, there is a pansystolic mitral murmur transmitted to the axilla and a diastolic mitral murmur of variable length. In patients with moderate mitral incompetence, the murmur may last until the end of diastole at rapid heart rates (more than 100/min.). The murmur is never accentuated during atrial systole because even if the patient is in sinus rhythm, the mitral stenosis is not sufficient to limit atrial emptying, and the force of contraction of the distended left atrium is reduced. In patients with atrial fibrillation, the length of the mitral diastolic murmur depends on the R-R interval of the preceding beat. A long diastolic pause allows time for equilibration between left atrial and left ventricular pressure. With long pauses, the murmur disappears towards the end of diastole. It is thus important to ascertain the length of the diastolic murmur during the longest pauses. In mixed mitral stenosis and incompetence, the murmur is less than full length at a normal heart rate of 70/min.

Pulmonary congestion in mixed mitral valve disease is less marked than in mitral stenosis. Although pulmonary edema may occur at the onset of atrial fibrillation, control of the heart rate by digitalis usually leads to rapid improvement, and the symptom seldom recurs. Similarly, an increase in pulmonary vascular resistance seldom occurs and is not often severe in mixed mitral valve disease, presumably, because left atrial pressure is lower than in pure stenosis. The most important factors to consider in mixed mitral valve disease are heart rate and heart rhythm. The whole clinical picture is greatly dependent on these factors and the efforts of changes in heart rate and rhythm. The whole clinical picture is greatly dependent on these factors, and the effects of changes in heart rate on the patient's condition offer the best means of assessing the severity of the lesion.

Differential Diagnosis

A. **Atrial Septal Defect:** Atrial septal defect with normal pulmonary vascular resistance and hypertrophic obstructive cardiomyopathy enter into the differential diagnosis of patients with mixed mitral stenosis and incompetence. In atrial septal defect, atrial fibrillation, cardiac enlargement, and systolic and diastolic murmurs occur, and in the middle-aged patient, an erroneous history of rheumatic fever in childhood is sometimes present. With these findings, the incorrect diagnosis of rheumatic heart disease is easily made. Radiologic examination is most useful because in atrial septal defect the chest X-ray shows a large pulmonary artery, a small aorta, a big heart, a big right atrium, and a left atrium that is usually unimpressive. The ECG almost invariably shows incomplete or complete right bundle block with an rsR' pattern in lead V1. This finding should always raise the suspicion that an atrial defect exists. Cardiac catheterization is ordinarily required to establish the diagnosis with certainty. The two lesions—mitral valve disease and atrial septal defect—may rarely coexist in Lutembacher's syndrome. In this condition, raised venous pressure, hepatomegaly, and peripheral edema are common, and the presence of right heart failure in a patient with mixed mitral stenosis and incompetence should always suggest an associated atrial septal defect.

B. **Hypertrophic Cardiomyopathy:** Patients with hypertrophic cardiomyopathy (who tend to be confused with those with mixed mitral valve disease) have lesions of the left ventricular inflow tract, with or without outflow obstruction. This lesion is rare, but when it is present mitral systolic and diastolic murmurs and mitral incompetence are seen. Significant left ventricular hypertrophy is always seen on the ECG. Echocardiography shows narrowing of the left ventricular outflow tract and systolic anterior motion of the aortic cusp of the mitral valve. Left ventricular catheterization and angiography are needed to confirm the diagnosis.

MITRAL INCOMPETENCE

Mitral incompetence differs from other forms of mitral valve disease in that it occurs as both an acute and a chronic lesion. The chronic lesions are further subdivided into hemodynamically insignificant and significant lesion. The hemodynamically insignificant form is present in those patients with the "click-murmur" syndrome described by Barlow, sometimes referred to as the floppy valve syndrome or mitral valve prolapse, but these terms are unsatisfactory because prolapse and "floppy valves" may cause acute mitral incompetence and imply a pathologic process that cannot be determined at the bedside.

Clinical Findings of Mitral Valve Prolapse (MVP)

1. **Symptoms**: Most patients are entirely symptom-free, and the condition is found accidentally on routine physical examination. In some cases, atypical chest pain is present, and palpitations, fatigue, and dyspnea unrelated to exertion also occur. Exercise tolerance is usually normal. Symptoms are more likely in patients who know they have the lesion. A family history of the lesion is occasionally found, and there may be a familial history of sudden death.
2. **Signs**: The only abnormalities are usually auscultatory in nature. The characteristic sign is a late systolic murmur. It is often preceded by one or more midsystolic clicks. The murmur increases in intensity up to the second heart sound, making it difficult to time and often leading to an incorrect diagnosis of diastolic murmur. It may become pansystolic with exercise or when the patient stands up. It often has a honking quality and may on occasion be loud enough to be heard without a stethoscope. It is not uncommonly the only abnormal finding and its timing is its most consistent feature. In some cases, a click is heard without a murmur. In such patients, mitral valve prolapse without mitral incompetence is thought to be present.

Differential Diagnosis Mitral Valve Prolapse

The physical signs of click-murmur syndrome are sufficiently specific to make the diagnosis of hemodynamically insignificant mitral

incompetence reasonably certain. The underlying pathology and the causes are more difficult to determine, however, and the significance of the lesion is always open to question. The presence of associated coronary artery disease may have to be ruled out by angiography in some cases.

Clinical Findings of Mitral Incompetence

Symptoms

1. **Acute lesions:** Dyspnea is the principal presenting symptom in patients with acute mitral incompetence. The onset may be acute, (e.g. when a cusp perforates or tears), or subacute (e.g. when the mitral valve gradually shrinks and retracts after treatment of endocarditis). Dyspnea may progress to acute pulmonary edema with acute circulatory collapse, shock, and frothy pink, blood-tinged sputum. The patient may be ill at the time of onset, with a high fever and septicemia. Episodic attacks of dyspnea may occur and are associated with minor increases in cardiac output in response to the exertion of meals, washing, bowel movements, or even the excitement of visitors. Left atrial pressure is markedly dependent on the peripheral resistance in this lesion, and any increase in arterial pressure may provoke an attack of dyspnea.
2. **Chronic lesions:** In hemodynamically significant lesions, dyspnea is the principal presenting symptom. It is not usually as severe as in mitral stenosis, and the effects of an increase in heart rate are less prominent. The onset of atrial fibrillation is generally well tolerated and does not provoke the acute symptoms seen in patients who have mitral stenosis. Palpitations are more common than in other forms of mitral disease; atrial fibrillation is the commonest cause. Patients do not usually present with symptoms due to systemic embolism, but such symptoms can occur, especially in the presence of endocarditis.

Signs

The first heart sound is usually buried in the pansystolic murmur, but there is never an opening snap. The presence of an opening snap indicates that significant rheumatic mitral stenosis is present. There is almost invariably a loud third heart sound associated with the rapid phase of left ventricular filling. It is a dull, low-pitched, thudding sound occurring about 0.10–0.18 second after the second sound. Some observers may consider it long enough to be called a diastolic murmur. Differences of opinion may arise about whether any degree of mitral stenosis is present. The characteristic murmur is a loud, high pitched, pansystolic apical murmur transmitted to the axilla. It is louder on expiration and decreases when systemic vascular resistance decreases acutely, as occurs with amyl nitrate inhalation.

Signs of right heart failure and raised pulmonary vascular resistance are rare except in patients with severe acute mitral incompetence resulting from acute disruption of the valve. The presence of right sided failure with increased venous pressure in a patient with mitral incompetence should suggest the possibility of associated organic tricuspid valve disease.

Differential Diagnosis of Mitral Incompetence

Mitral incompetence must be distinguished from hypertrophic cardiomyopathy. There is a long pansystolic murmur in both conditions, and although the murmur in mitral incompetence is usually higher pitched, has a timing that is not of the ejection type, and is transmitted to the axilla rather than centrally, the two lesions can be confused on diagnosis. Both show a third heart sound and a prominent left ventricle.

Ventricular septal defect is another condition that can be confused with mitral incompetence. Again, the auscultatory findings are similar, with an overactive left ventricle, a pansystolic murmur, and third heart sound. Chest X-ray may be helpful if the ventricular septal defect is large enough to cause increased lung markings resulting from increased pulmonary blood flow, but even these markings can be confused with those due to pulmonary congestion. Endocardial cushion defects with an associated ostium primum atrial defect and mitral incompetence are also difficult to differentiate from pure mitral incompetence and cardiac catheterization is almost invariably needed to confirm the diagnosis. In the case of acute lesions, especially in patients who have suffered a recent myocardial infarction, the distinction between acquired ventricular septal defect due to rupture of the ventricular septum and acute mitral incompetence due to papillary muscle involvement can be extremely difficult. Here, too, as in all significant lesions, cardiac catheterization and angiography are necessary to confirm the diagnosis before surgery.

■ AORTIC VALVE DISEASE

It is tolerated rather well for a long time as compared to mitral disease. Aortic valve disease is the next most common form of valvular heart disease after mitral disease and accounts for about 35% of patients with significant valvular lesions. Classification is difficult because of the varied causes, hemodynamic severity, acuteness or chronicity, anatomic site and nature of the lesion.

Classification

Aortic valve disease has been classified in this text into three main categories; (1) hemodynamically insignificant aortic valve disease, (2) hemodynamically significant predominant aortic incompetence, and (3) hemodynamically significant predominant aortic incompetence.

In hemodynamically insignificant aortic value disease, it is impossible to determine whether stenosis or incompetence is predominant because the lesion is so mild. There is no evidence of cardiac enlargement or hypertrophy and no limitation of exercise tolerance. It is not possible to predict whether the lesion will progress, or if it does, whether aortic stenosis or aortic incompetence will predominate.

Hemodynamically significant aortic valve disease accompanying other forms of heart disease such as hypertension, atherosclerosis, or disease of other valves complicates the classification. In such cases, complete investigation is often needed to confirm the diagnosis; the existence of predominant aortic stenosis is often suspected before left heart catheterization is performed, and the correct diagnosis is not established until the investigations have been completed.

Hemodynamically aortic valve lesions from pure stenosis through mixed stenosis and incompetence to pure incompetence. It is thus difficult to know how to separate patients into groups for the purposes of classification. Because aortic stenosis is a more serious lesion than aortic incompetence, the lesions of all patients with any element of stenosis are classified as predominantly stenotic rather incompetence.

An indirectly recorded brachial arterial diastolic blood pressure of 70 mm Hg or more is used as arbitrary measurement below which hemodynamically significant aortic incompetence is present. This cutoff is naturally not entirely satisfactory, but it represents the best single figure on which the classification is based. In practice, the level of the systolic arterial pressure, the rate of rise of the carotid pulse, the pulse pressure, the quality of the left ventricular impulse, the degree of left ventricular hypertrophy, and the presence of absence of left ventricular failure all assist the cardiologist in determining whether the lesion is predominantly stenotic or incompetent and whether it is hemodynamically significant or not.

Acute and Chronic Aortic Incompetence

Aortic incompetence, like mitral incompetence, occurs in both the acute and the chronic forms. Acute lesions are almost always due to the effects of infective endocarditis but may rarely occur when acute aortic dissection involves the aortic root. The acute load on the left ventricle causes a clinical picture that is different from that seen in chronic lesions. Acute left ventricular failure with severe pulmonary congestion and edema can occur within a few hours or days, and the lesion is often fatal if valve replacement is not performed. The degree of acuteness varies from case to case. Some of the most severe lesions are seen when an aortic cusp is form or perforated. In acute aortic incompetence, the patient's condition seldom stabilizes without valve replacement, but in a few cases in which the onset is less acute, the changes associated with chronic aortic incompetence—left ventricular hypertrophy and dilatation—develop over several weeks, and after a year, the clinical picture is indistinguishable from that seen in chronic aortic incompetence.

Causes of Aortic Valve Lesions

To detect both the cause and severity of aortic valve lesions is difficult by ordinary clinical means. There is often a discrepancy between the patient's symptoms and the hemodynamic severity of the lesions, and the cause often remains in doubt, even after autopsy. Both aortic stenosis and aortic incompetence may run long clinical courses lasting 20–30 years, and the physician is often confronted with patients who have hemodynamically significant lesions and yet no symptoms. Just as frequently, the patient has symptoms that are out of proportion to the hemodynamic findings. Because aortic valve lesions can run such a long clinical course, it is difficult to determine what factors are responsible for the progressive deterioration of the patient's clinical state that often occurs over a short period of a few weeks or months. Long-term changes may be due to valvular calcification or myocardial fibrosis, but the patient nonetheless suddenly develops left ventricular failure, and the disease runs a rapid downhill course that is not always reversed by surgical treatment.

As in mitral valve disease, rheumatic fever is an important cause of aortic valvular lesions. A history of previous rheumatic fever is present in 20% of patients with predominant stenosis and in 25% of those with predominant incompetence. Since congenital aortic valve lesions are relatively common, some patients who have been diagnosed as having had rheumatic fever in childhood actually have congenital aortic valve lesions. Seventy five percent of patients with predominant aortic stenosis who have a past history of rheumatic fever are women, whereas 75% of those with pure incompetence who have a past history of rheumatic fever are men. This agrees with the finding in mitral valve disease that stenosis occurs more commonly in females and incompetence in males. Aortic valve disease is more prevalent in males by a factor of 3:1 in predominant stenosis and 3:2 in predominant incompetence. These proportions vary in different series for the reason that causes vary in different geographic areas.

Hemodynamically Insignificant Lesions

The cardinal features of hemodynamically insignificant aortic lesions include normal heart size and hemodynamics and a systolic ejection murmur. The variable features are a systolic ejection click and a short aortic diastolic murmur. Auscultatory physical signs arising from the aortic valve are usually the sole abnormality. These lesions constitute 10% of cases seen in university hospital practice but make up a much larger percentage in private practice. These cases probably represent a presymptomatic phase of aortic valve disease that if followed long enough would be seen in develop into either aortic stenosis or aortic incompetence. The most important complication in such cases is the development of infective endocarditis, with associated development or exacerbation of aortic incompetence. These lesions are seen in patients of all ages. Congenital, rheumatic, and atherosclerotic causes account for two-thirds of cases; no causative factor is identified in the others.

Clinical Features

More than half of cases are entirely asymptomatic. In the others, palpitations, fatigue, dizziness, and non-cardiac dyspnea occur but without evidence of heart failure. Symptoms are more common in patients who are aware that they have a heart murmur. The pulse and blood pressure are normal; a collapsing pulse or a slow-rising pulse is, by definition, absent. The heart is not enlarged on clinical or X-ray examination, and no evidence of ventricular hypertrophy is detectable. (If any of these signs are present, the lesion is no longer hemodynamically insignificant). There is always a systolic murmur at the base of the heart, preceded by an ejection click in one-third of cases and followed by a faint aortic diastolic murmur in one-third. Slight aortic dilation is occasionally seen, but valvular calcification is not necessarily present.

Cardiac catheterization is not indicated for diagnosis, but if it is performed, intracardiac pressures are normal, and there is no significant pressure difference between the left ventricle and the aorta. Such patients can subsequently develop predominant aortic stenosis, but the course in individual cases is difficult to predict. Long-term follow-up of 20 years or more is often necessary.

The role of the deposition of calcium in these slightly abnormal valves is difficult to determine, but it seems likely that valvular calcification immobilizes and narrows the valve, causing stenosis that gradually progresses but does not significantly load the left ventricle until the valve is narrowed to about one-fourth its normal area $(5.0 \text{ cm}^2 \longrightarrow 1.25 \text{ cm}^2)$.

The other important development in such cases is infective endocarditis. Patients with hemodynamically insignificant aortic lesions are particularly prone to this complication, and the valve is likely to become acutely and severely incompetent as a result. Thus, the prevention and early recognition of endocarditis are important aspects of the management of patients with this lesion. Antibiotic prophylactic therapy preceding major dental work or minor surgery and early blood culture during febrile illnesses is mandatory. Intravenous drug abuse is particularly likely to result in infective endocarditis because contaminated needles and syringes are often used, and the drugs are seldom sterile. When a rheumatic origin for the lesion is suspected, prophylactic penicillin treatment is warranted to prevent recurrences of rheumatic fever.

Predominant Aortic Stenosis

The cardinal features of predominant aortic stenosis are left ventricular hypertrophy and a systolic ejection murmur. The variable factors are the severity, which affects the hypertrophy; the site of the obstruction; the cause; and the presence or absence of valvular calcification.

Importance of Aortic Stenosis

Predominant aortic stenosis has an importance in clinical cardiology that is out of proportion to its frequency. The reason for this is that both the diagnosis and the assessment of severity of the lesion are often extremely difficult. Aortic stenosis is easily missed on clinical examination, especially if the patient is in severe left ventricular failure and the cardiac output is so low that the aortic systolic murmur that might point toward a diagnosis of aortic stenosis is virtually inaudible. Aortic stenosis is often suspected in patients in whom there is no significant obstruction to aortic flow. In these cases, it is the presence of an aortic systolic murmur, often associated with calcification of the aortic valve on fluoroscopy that indicates possible aortic stenosis. Although echocardiography may be valuable in ruling out a diagnosis of aortic stenosis, left heart catheterization is always indicated to confirm that obstruction is severe. Approximately, 10% of patients undergoing cardiac catheterization in a university hospital subsequently prove to have hemodynamically unimportant lesions despite a diagnosis of aortic stenosis before

the procedure, but the risks of missing the correct catheterization that the study should be performed if there is the slightest doubt about the diagnosis.

Cause of Aortic Stenosis

The cause of aortic stenosis has been the subject of controversy for many years. In most cases (70%), there is no clinical clue to the cause. At autopsy, the valve is usually so disorganized by calcification that it is difficult to count the number of cusps. Now that aortic valve replacement has become routine, the valve is available for study at an earlier stage of the disease, and it is easier to see if there are two or three cusps. Even so, separate cusps cannot be identified in some patients (15%). Since the normal aortic valve has three cusps, the findings of a bicuspid valve in 50% of patients indicates that the basic lesion is congenital in patients with predominant aortic stenosis who undergo surgery or die of the disease. Patients with bicuspid valves often have other congenital lesion, most commonly coarctation of the aorta. Some are known to have had a murmur since early infancy, but the majority (2/3) have had a murmur first heard only after age 20. This latter group generally does not have congenital aortic stenosis but rather a minor congenital valvular lesion that apparently makes the valve more than normally susceptible to wear and tear.

Congenital aortic stenosis is rarely seen in adults and constitutes about 5% of cases. In such cases, a murmur has almost always been heart in infancy, and symptoms usually have developed in early adult life. All patients with predominant aortic stenosis tend to develop valvular calcification with increasing age, and after age 40, valvular calcification is present in virtually all cases, irrespective of the cause of the lesion. Age-related degenerative changes in the valve thus seem to be important in the progression of the lesion.

In a small but increasing number of patients, atherosclerotic, age-related degenerative changes in a normal valve appear to be the sole cause of aortic stenosis. In this group, the valve is tricuspid, the patient is over age 60, and a murmur has not been present for more than 5 years. This group of patients constitutes about 10% of cases. There is some suggestion that aortic stenosis may develop rapidly in such patients and run a shorter course. Associated coronary artery disease is common in this group.

Clinical Findings

In all forms of aortic stenosis, a fixed, disorganized, calcified, thickened, radiopaque mass of tissue replaces the normal flexible, thin, filmy valve structure. In congenital aortic stenosis, the valve is often dome-shaped, and no cusps can be distinguished. Calcification is most closely related to age and occurs at the earliest in the late teens and 20s. The development of calcification is commonly associated with the development of an aortic systolic ejection murmur.

Aortic stenosis increases the work of the left ventricle. In cases of pure stenosis, hypertrophy first occurs at the expense of the left ventricular cavity, causing a decrease in ventricular compliance. The ventricle becomes more rounded, but overall heart size is not increased. If there is associated aortic incompetence, the left ventricle is larger, and in most cases, heart size is increased by the time symptoms appear. The narrowing of the aortic valve produces turbulence and often causes a jet stream of blood to impinge on the anterior and right walls of the aorta, resulting in a localized, poststenotic dilatation of the aorta. The calcification of the aortic valve may spread to the valve ring and thence to the anterior (aortic) cusp of the mitral valve and the membranous part of the interventricular conduction defects. The coronary vessels are usually large and not atherosclerotic and younger patients with bicuspid valves, but calcific emboli may occur and cause coronary occlusion or other serious systemic embolism. Aortic stenosis developing de novo in elderly persons is more likely to be associated with coronary artery disease, and the combination carries a poor prognosis.

Blood is subject to extremely severe mechanical stress as it passed through the turbulent area associated with a stenotic aortic valve. Damage to red cells in the form of excessive hemolysis may occur in patients with aortic stenosis, especially if the cells are abnormally fragile. This rare form of hemolytic anemia is also seen after aortic valve replacement.

A. **Symptoms:** Symptoms appear late in the course of aortic stenosis, and many patients with hemodynamically significant lesions have no complaints. The disease is not recognized in its earlier stages, usually because the patient does not seek medical advice. In some cases, the murmur has been present without any symptoms for so many years that the physician overlooks the possibility of aortic stenosis until it becomes severe.

The stage at which symptoms develop depends to some extent on the patient's activity level. In sedentary people, the disease may be far advanced before the patient complains of symptoms. Half of patients with surgically significant aortic stenosis have had at least one episode of left ventricular failure before they undergo surgery for stenosis. In active persons, dyspnea on exertion occurs before overt left ventricular failure develops, but especially in sedentary people, an episode of paroxysmal nocturnal dyspnea may be the first symptom of disease.

That aortic stenosis runs a long pre-symptomatic course is evident from the finding that significant stenosis—as judged by the presence of a systolic murmur and left ventricular hypertrophy on the ECG—may be present for 20 years without causing any symptoms. The course of the disease after symptoms' development is rapid. Progressive left ventricular failure leads to death in 2–8 years, if surgery is not performed. The symptoms in the later stages of aortic stenosis are some of the most difficult to manage in the entire spectrum of cardiac disease. Nightly attacks of paroxysmal dyspnea, with sweating, collapse, extreme restlessness, and intractable shortness of breath, cause severe distress. Morphine and potent diuretics are the drugs of choice in the medical management of such patients, but physicians who have had to treat patients at this stage of the disease tend to favor surgical treatment for all patients with significant aortic stenosis, regardless of age.

Dyspnea on exertion is the commonest presenting symptom (75% of cases) in predominant aortic stenosis. As in other forms of left ventricular overload, shortness of breath is quantitatively related to exertion and is often accompanied by a heavy, tight feeling in the chest that is discomfort rather than pain and is only perceived in association with dyspnea. This sensation may occasionally radiate to the arms and is often interpreted as angina pectoris. Dyspnea on effort ordinarily precedes the episodes of paroxysmal nocturnal dyspnea, which herald the onset of left ventricular failure. Dizziness (10% of patients) and cardiac pain (10%) are the next most common presenting symptoms of aortic stenosis; syncope on unaccustomed effort is the other principal symptom. It occurs in about 5% of cases, usually early in the disease before the left ventricle has failed. In many patients, it only occurs once, because the patient associates the syncope with over-exertion and subsequently avoids lifting heavy objects, shoveling snow, running upstairs, or performing whatever activity precipitated the first attack. Loss of consciousness is usually preceded by dyspnea, which the patient disregards, perhaps because of the circumstances surrounding the over-exertion. Recovery from the syncopal attack is rapid, and sudden death, which is common in aortic stenosis, seldom occurs on exertion. It is of great importance to obtain a clear history of the circumstances surrounding a syncopal episode in a patient suspected of having aortic stenosis. If syncope is provoked only by severe effort, stenosis is already severe. Syncope unrelated to excessive effort is more common than effort syncope in aortic stenosis (10%) but is not necessarily an indication that severe stenosis is present. Such syncope is often due to arrhythmia rather than an inadequate increase in cardiac output during stress. It is often confused with transient cerebral ischemic attacks due to atherosclerosis of the cerebral vessels in patients who have aortic systolic murmurs but no aortic stenosis.

Cardiac pain in patients with aortic stenosis is attributed either to failure of coronary blood flow to meet the increased demands of the hypertrophied left ventricular myocardium or to associated coronary disease in older patients. It is important to distinguish two types of cardiac pain in aortic stenosis. The commonest form is a heavy substernal discomfort, described as a bursting, choking, constricting feeling that only comes when the patient is dyspneic. It may occur more readily after meals and radiate to the arms, but it never occurs without dyspnea. It differs from true angina of effort, in which the pain or discomfort is clearly the primary event and occurs before dyspnea. If both of these forms of cardiac distress are termed angina, then the commonest symptom of aortic stenosis is indeed angina. However, if the term angina is reserved for pain that is not associated with or preceded by dyspnea, then angina is the presenting symptom of only 10% of patients with aortic stenosis.

B. **Signs**: The arterial pulse in patients with predominant aortic stenosis is of small amplitude and is slow-rising because left ventricular ejection time through the narrowed aortic valve is prolonged. Such an arterial pulse is termed as anacrotic pulse, plateau pulse, or pulsus tardus, because the wave takes longer than normal to pass beneath the examiner's fingers. The examiner should also feel the radial, brachial, femoral, and carotid pulses. The carotid pulse, being closest to the aortic valve, gives the most accurate information. The rise time is slowed and the time taken to reach peak pressure is increased in the central pulse in aortic stenosis. Pressure tracings may show an anacrotic notch on the upstroke; the lower on the upstroke it occurs, the more severe the lesion. In patients with mixed lesion in whom there is also aortic incompetence, the upstroke of the pulse is more rapid, and a double peaked pulse (pulsus bisferiens) may be found. Pulsus bisferiens is more likely to be present in a more peripheral artery (e.g. radial or brachial) and is not usually seen in the central aortic pulse. The presence of pulsus bisferiens is not of diagnostic significance. Before aortic valve replacement was available, pulsus bisferiens was taken as evidence that aortic incompetence was too severe to warrant aortic valvotomy. This operation like mitral valvotomy, tended to convert pure stenosis to mixed stenosis and incompetence.

Blood pressure is ordinarily low, with a narrow pulse pressure, and reflects the small stroke volume in aortic stenosis. However, it may be normal, especially in patients with mixed lesions. Systemic hypertension, although uncommon, does not rule out surgically significant aortic stenosis. An a wave may be seen in the jugular venous pulse if the ventricular septum bulges to the right and impairs right ventricular filling, or if severe pulmonary hypertension develops. The heart rate is usually regular, but about 10% of patients are in atrial fibrillation at the time of surgery. The incidence of atrial fibrillation in cases with a history of rheumatic fever is no greater than in those with congenitally bicuspid aortic valves, but atrial fibrillation should always alert the physician to the possibility of coexisting associated mitral valve disease. The

degree of left ventricular hypertrophy on physical examination—as shown by the prominence of the left ventricular heave—depends on the severity and purity of the stenosis. If the chest wall is thin, a left ventricular heave is readily seen and felt, but in many patients, it is necessary to rely on the ECG for evidence of left ventricular hypertrophy. The degree of left ventricular enlargement on physical examination depends largely on the degree of aortic incompetence accompanying the aortic stenosis. The examining hand readily perceives the dynamic quality of the ventricular impulse, which primarily reflects left ventricular stroke volume. The degree of left ventricular enlargement is better detected on the chest X-ray than on physical examination, especially when left ventricular failure has reduced the stroke volume.

Since in most cases the aortic valve is thickened, immobilized by calcification, and stenotic, it does not close properly, and some degree of aortic incompetence, the larger the heart. Predominant aortic stenosis varies from cases with no incompetence to those with an aortic leak sufficient to give a normal or slightly widened pulse pressure and a slightly hyperdynamic left ventricular impulse.

Depending on the anatomy of the valve, an aortic valve closure sound may or may not be present. If A_2 is audible, paradoxical (reversed) splitting of the second heart sound may be heard, if severe stenosis or left bundle branch block is present. Third and fourth heart sounds are commonly heard. The characteristic murmur of aortic stenosis is harsh and chugging, and its timing is ejection in nature, starting after isometric contraction has occurred, i.e. 0.06 second or more after the first heart sound. It is usually associated with a systolic thrill at the base. It is preceded by an ejection click only in mild cases, when the aortic valve is more flexible and ventricular ejection more rapid. The murmur may be heard at the base or the apex of the heart. It is often heard well in the neck, but this does not mean it is aortic in origin, since pulmonary systolic murmurs and bruits of carotid artery stenosis are also well heard there. The murmur starts after the first heart sound and stop before the second heart sound. It is louder after a long pause following an ectopic beat, and it varies with cardiac filling in atrial fibrillation. It may be audible only at the apex of the heart and can be easily missed if the patient is in severe left ventricular failure. A faint aortic diastolic murmur along the left sternal edge is usually present, but its loudness does not necessarily correspond to the severity of associated aortic incompetence, which is judge instead by the character of the pulse, the size of the heart, and the dynamic qualities of the left ventricular impulse.

Rales at the base of the lungs are heard in patients with left ventricular failure, and signs of right ventricular failure with raised jugular venous pressure, hepatomegaly, and peripheral edema are late manifestations of the disease. They are generally due to the development of a raised pulmonary vascular resistance (> 3.5 mm Hg/min), which occurs in a small proportion (about 10%) of cases.

Diagnosis

The most pressing problems in the diagnosis of aortic stenosis are; (1) to detect when left ventricular failure will occur in the course of the disease, (2) to assess accurately the severity of stenosis, and (3) to decide whether to recommend surgery for asymptomatic and mildly symptomatic patients. The presence of left ventricular hypertrophy on the ECG or physical examination may raise the possibility of surgery but is not an absolute indication for further clinical investigation, since a patient with the disease can be asymptomatic for up to 20 years with moderate left ventricular hypertrophy.

On the other hand, the possibility that dyspnea, syncope, dizziness, or cardiac pain is due to aortic stenosis is a strong indication for left heart catheterization. Echocardiography can reduce the number of patients in whom cardiac catheterization is performed by showing that the aortic valve is thin and mobile. The physician must maintain a strong index of suspicion and a sense of urgency in dealing with patients whose symptoms may be due to aortic stenosis, because delay is more dangerous in aortic stenosis than in any other cardiac lesion in adults. There is no substitute for left heart catheterization as a means of determining the severity of obstruction; physical signs, an ECG, presence of aortic valve calcification, aortic angiography, and the shape or movement of the valve on echocardiography are all incapable of providing consistently correct assessments of severity, although they may lead to a correct diagnosis in 85% of cases. Color Doppler is now a better choice.

Differential Diagnosis

A. **Left Ventricular Failure**: Aortic stenosis enters into the differential diagnosis of all patients with left ventricular failure, especially when there is a basal systolic murmur and a history of syncope, dizziness, or conduction defect. The possibility of aortic stenosis must be considered in hypertension, cardiomyopathy, and even in coronary artery disease, especially when heart failure is severe. It is important to recognize the systolic murmur and rule out the possibility of aortic stenosis by all available means, including cardiac catheterization. In many centers, all patients with cardiomyopathy undergo cardiac catheterization in order to rule out aortic stenosis.

B. **Hypertrophic Obstruction Cardiomyopathy**: Aortic stenosis should not be confused with hypertrophic obstructive cardiomyopathy. In the latter condition, the pulse is jerky and the upstroke rapid and often bifid, in contrast to the slow-rising pulse of aortic stenosis. If there is associated aortic incompetence modifying the upstroke of the pulse in a patient with predominant aortic stenosis, there will almost certainly be an aortic diastolic murmur, which virtually rules out a diagnosis of obstructive cardiomyopathy is longer, harsher and usually heard best to the left of the sternum. The variation occurring in the murmur when diagnostic measures are used to influence the extent of outflow tract narrowing is helpful in establishing the diagnosis of obstructive cardiomyopathy. Echocardiography is particularly helpful in differential diagnosis because it shows systolic anterior motion of the mitral valve in hypertrophic cardiomyopathy and aortic valve thickening in aortic stenosis. Left heart catheterization and left ventricular angiography were generally used to confirm the diagnosis, now color Doppler is preferred.

C. **Other Lesions**: The physical signs in mitral incompetence and ventricular septal defect are seldom confused with those of predominant aortic stenosis. In these disorders, the murmur is pansystolic, and the carotid upstroke is rapid. When the patient has both aortic stenosis and mitral incompetence, it is difficult to distinguish between them, and clinical assessment of the relative severity of the two lesions is usually impossible. In some cases, there is a characteristic high pitched "seagull cry" murmur.

Coarctation of the aorta is another lesion, which may occasionally coexist with aortic stenosis and be confused with it. The murmur of coarctation occurs later in systole and reaches its peak about the time of the second heart sound. There is characteristically a prominent carotid arterial pulsation as well as delay between the peaks of the branchial and femoral pulses, with hypertension in the arms. Although coarctation of the aorta is commonly associated with bicuspid aortic valve, the coarctation is likely to cause problems long before the abnormal valve gives rise to difficulties that are associated with the development of aortic stenosis resulting from calcification of the abnormal valve.

Predominant Aortic Incompetence

The cardinal features of hemodynamically significant predominant aortic incompetence include a large hypertrophied left ventricle, a large aorta, increased stroke volume, and wide pulse pressure. Variable factors include the severity of the process, the nature of the lesion (acute or chronic), and the cause.

Hemodynamically significant aortic incompetence creates an important extra load on the left ventricle. The blood that flows back across the aortic valve during diastole must be ejected during systole, and the consequent large stroke volume increases the work of the heart. The extra work is mainly "flow" work rather than "pressure" work, but peak systolic pressure tends to be raised and aortic diastolic pressure lowered because of rapid runoff of aortic blood into the peripheral arterial bed and back into the left ventricle. The arbitrary basis on which aortic incompetence is classified as hemodynamically significant here is the level of diastolic pressure. A value to less than 70 mm Hg. constitutes the dividing line, and patients with aortic incompetence and arterial diastolic pressure higher than that are generally considered to have hemodynamically insignificant aortic incompetence. Exceptions do exist, especially in patients in severe heart failure, in whom peripheral vasoconstriction has occurred and caused an increased diastolic pressure.

Acute Lesions

Aortic incompetence occurs both as an acute lesion (20% of cases) and as a single chronic lesion (80% of cases). Acute aortic incompetence occurs when valve lesion develop either instantaneously—when a cusp perforates or tears—or over a few days or weeks—when valve tissue is gradually eroded by infection, or when fibrosis, associated with healing of an infection, scars and contracts the valve. Acute aortic incompetence throws a more serious load on the left ventricle than acute mitral incompetence, and the chances that the patient's hemodynamic status will stabilize without surgical treatment are small. If the damage is less severe or less acute, the possibility for survival is better; and if the patient survives, the clinical picture in acute aortic incompetence by the end of about one year resembles that in chronic lesions. The hemodynamic load in acute lesions tends to fall mainly on the lungs, and acute left ventricular failure usually develops before left ventricular hypertrophy or dilatation has had time to occur. If the patient has marked pulmonary edema, the peripheral signs of aortic incompetence, with wide pulse pressure and low diastolic pressure, may be masked because arteriolar vasoconstriction has occurred in response to impaired perfusion, but there should still be an obvious aortic diastolic murmur.

Chronic Lesions

Chronic aortic incompetence results in marked peripheral vasodilatation, which is attributable in part to reflex baroreceptor effect. The wide aortic and carotid pulse pressure cause reflex vasodilatation and relative bradycardia. With exercise, the cardiac output increases, there is peripheral vasodilatation of the muscular capillaries, and a further fall in systemic vascular resistance occurs. As a result, the proportion of the left ventricular stroke volume returning to the left ventricle during diastole falls, and the hemodynamic status becomes closer to that seen in normal subjects. In contrast, anything that increases the systemic vascular resistance, such as isometric exercise, exposure to cold, sympathetic nervous system stimulation, mental stress, or cardiac failure, tends to increase the volume of blood returning to the ventricle during diastole and makes the load on the heart more a "pressure" load and less a "flow" load.

Clinical Findings

In rheumatic lesions, fibrosis and retraction of the valve cusps start early in the course of rheumatic infection and progress slowly over several years. Syphilis attacked the aortic valve secondarily, by extension of disease from the aorta. Endarteritis obliterans of the vasa vasorum of the aorta is the basic pathologic lesion of syphilitic aortitis, and aortic dilatation with swelling and thickening of the intima involves the root of the aorta and perhaps the coronary ostia, leading to myocardial ischemia. In congenital lesions, the valve lesion is often secondary to aortic dilatation, as in Marfan's syndrome, or to prolapse of unsupported valvular tissue, as in association with ventricular septal defects involving the membranous part of the interventricular septum. There is no associated myocarditis in congenital cases; as a result, muscle damage is less prominent. In ankylosing spondylitis and Reiter's syndrome, the pathologic lesion is again primarily in the aorta and in the connective tissues supporting the valve. In atherosclerotic lesions, too, it is aortic involvement that secondarily affects the valve, principally by means of dilatation.

A. Symptoms:
1. **Acute lesions**: Dyspnea is the commonest presenting cardiac symptom in acute lesions (50% of cases). Since infective endocarditis is by far the commonest cause, the patient usually is febrile and may be acutely ill with septicemia at the time that the aortic valve lesion develops. In other cases, the onset is slower and subacute: the aortic lesion appears or worsens as endocarditis heals, and the valve shrinks as it fibroses weeks or months after the endocarditis has responded to antibiotic therapy. In other patients, systemic embolism may be the presenting symptom, with a cerebrovascular accident, an acute coronary occlusion, or a cold, painful leg as the first sign of acute aortic incompetence. Acute aortic incompetence occurring in a person who is not ill with infective endocarditis suggests the possibility of acute aortic dissection involving the noncoronary cusp of the aortic valve. This uncommon lesion is not always painful, if either the left or right coronary artery is involved, the patient almost inevitably dies.

    The dyspnea of acute aortic incompetence is often paroxysmal and associated with orthopnea and cough, with frothy pink sputum resulting from acute pulmonary edema. Chest pain may occur because of acute myocardial ischemia and peripheral circulatory collapse. Symptoms of shock, with anxiety, confusion, and mental obtundation are occasionally seen.

2. **Chronic lesions:**

   a. **Symptoms unrelated to severity:** There are two varieties of symptoms in chromic aortic incompetence, those due to the patient's awareness of increased force of the heart beat and those due to left ventricular disease and heart failure. One-third of patients with hemodynamically significant aortic incompetence not infrequently complain of palpitations, which on questioning turn out to be associated with sensations arising from forceful left ventricular contraction. The patient often notices the symptoms when lying in bed at night. These sensations sometimes provoke the symptoms of anxiety seen in cardiac neurosis, with stabbing inframammary pain, fatigue, and dyspnea with sighing respirations. The patient may have ventricular premature beats that further accentuate the symptoms. These symptoms usually occur in early adult life and can be present for 20 years or more without significant progression of the valvular lesion. More frequently (two-thirds of cases), the patient has no symptoms and is able to lead a surprisingly normal, active life in spite of a hemodynamically serious lesion. It is important to recognize certain symptoms as "functional" in patients with aortic incompetence and not interpret them as a necessary indication for surgery. Ventricular

arrhythmia is probably the most important cause of symptoms at this stage, since it is though that it may precede ventricular tachycardia or fibrillation and these developments may account for the sudden death that is rarer in aortic incompetence than in stenosis but which nevertheless occurs. The presence of symptoms in a patient with aortic incompetence is always an indication for thorough investigation; but if the valvular lesion is well tolerated, the patient (especially if young) should usually simply be closely followed, and the physician should watch for the development of more serious symptoms.

   b. **Symptoms of left ventricular failure:** When aortic incompetence is the sole lesion, serious symptoms due to left ventricular failure occur late in the course of the disease. Dyspnea is by far the commonest symptom (75% of cases) and may be associated with a feeling of heaviness in the chest and substernal discomfort. If significant dyspnea occurs before age 30 and left ventricular failure is found, it is most likely that past or present rheumatic myocardial involvement is influencing the clinical picture. Left ventricular failure due solely to chronic aortic incompetence usually occurs after age 40, and patients who lead sedentary lives may not be aware of the insidious progression of pulmonary congestion because they have never exerted themselves sufficiently. In these patients, an acute episode of paroxysmal nocturnal dyspnea or frank pulmonary edema may be the presenting event. Chest pain is the next most common symptom in aortic incompetence. It is particularly common in patients with syphilitic lesions and in older persons with associated coronary arterial disease. Anginal pain may be present at rest or during exercise; in general, it is due to increased metabolic demands of the hypertrophied myocardium rather than to decreased supply resulting from obstructive atherosclerotic lesions in major coronary vessels. Syncope and dizziness are less common that in patients with predominantly stenotic lesions, and syncope during unaccustomed effort (the type seen in aortic stenosis) does not occur.

c. **Development of left ventricular failure**: The late symptoms in aortic incompetence carry a poor prognosis. This is in part due to reflex factors that cause a vicious circle. When cardiac output falls as the left ventricle fails, the normal peripheral vasodilatation seen in aortic incompetence is replaced by vasoconstriction because the carotid and aortic baroreceptors no longer transmit inhibitory sensory information via the glossopharyngeal nerve. This peripheral vasoconstriction increases the work of the left ventricle, increases aortic incompetence, and aggravates left ventricular failure. The relatively high arterial diastolic pressure that results may mislead the physician into thinking that significant aortic incompetence is not present. Left ventricular failure is thus especially sudden in aortic incompetence and is often provoked by factors involving autonomic nervous system control of blood pressure and blood volume, such as excitement, excessive sodium intake, recumbency, overexertion, excessive mental stress, and violent dreams, all of which cause a rise in systemic arterial pressure. The patient's occupation may also influence the occurrence of left ventricular failure. Patients with strenuous jobs involving heavy manual labor may develop larger hearts corresponding to a given level of severity in the lesion and hence develop left ventricular failure earlier than patients who avoid excessive exertion. The role of mental stress may also be important in patients with this lesion, because it is increased systemic arterial pressure and increased peripheral resistance that tend to aggravate incompetence more than any increase in cardiac output.

d. **Sweating**: Patients with predominant aortic incompetence have a tendency to sweat more, a finding that is unexplained. The mechanism is thought to involve the cholinergic sympathetic vasodilator fibers and be in some way elated to the wide pulse pressure, since a similar tendency is seen in other high output states such as thyrotoxicosis and Paget's disease.

B. **Signs**: The rapid runoff of blood from the aorta during diastole dominates the physical signs of hemodynamically significant aortic incompetence. Prominent carotid pulsations in the neck, throbbing peripheral arteries, and a prominent left ventricular impulse that moves the whole left side of the chest produce easily visible evidence of the large left ventricular stroke volume and increased rate of systolic ejection seen in this lesion. These peripheral circulatory signs are seen in both acute and chronic lesions and are present in all patients except those in severe left ventricular failure. The rapid aortic runoff is due to increased blood flow back into the left ventricle and into the dilated peripheral arterial bed. It is important to remember that rapid runoff from the aorta into cardiac chambers or blood vessels other than the left ventricle are an equally potent cause of the peripheral signs ordinarily associated with aortic incompetence. Large patent ductus arteriosus, aortopulmonary window rupture of an aneurysm of the aortic sinus (sinus of Valsalva) with consequent left-to-right shunt, or a major systemic arteriovenous fistula may produce similar physical signs.

Systemic arterial pressure is the most readily measured indication of the severity of the peripheral signs of rapid aortic runoff. There is a wide pulse pressure, with high systolic and low diastolic pressure. Arterial pressure measured indirectly with a blood pressure cuff is not always accurate, and a diastolic pressure reading of zero, indicating that there is an audible sound over the artery with no cuff in position, is never an accurate physical finding although it is often seen in patients with aortic incompetence. The wide pulse pressure gives rise to the typical collapsing pulse in which the pulse wave rises rapidly to a peak and falls away quickly. Secondary physical signs due to rapid aortic runoff are numerous and usually have eponymic designations. Head movement in time with the heartbeat is called Musset's sign after the French poet Alfred de Musset, in whom it was noticed by his brother, who was physician. Quincke's pulse denotes capillary pulsation in the extremities; Durozier's sign refers to systolic and diastolic murmurs over the femoral artery; and Hill's sign denotes increased blood pressure in the legs above that measured in the arms. Corrigan' s pulse refers to the collapsing pulse, which is also called a "water-hammer" pulse after a 19th century children's toy of that name (Fig. 2.5A and B). Pulsations in the digital and ulnar arteries are readily felt, and the hands and feet are warm and sweaty.

It is important to remember that rapid aortic runoff is a nonspecific clinical finding. Pulsation can also be seen in the second and third intercostal spaces to the right of the sternum when the aorta is dilated, especially in syphilitic lesions with or without associated aortic aneurysm. It is seen best from the side of the bed, with the examiner's eye at chest level.

In chronic aortic incompetence, the left ventricular impulse is hyperdynamic, and the apex beat is displaced downward and to the left. These physical signs depend largely on the size of the heart and are less obvious in acute aortic incompetence in which left ventricular hypertrophy has not yet developed. The characteristic physical sign on auscultation is a high-pitched, blowing diastolic murmur beginning immediately after the second sound at the start of diastole. It is called an "immediate" or early diastolic murmur to distinguish it from the "delayed" diastolic murmur of mitral stenosis, which does not start until left ventricular pressure has fallen below the level of left atrial pressure, ie, about 0.1 second after the start of diastole. The diastolic murmur of aortic incompetence lasts until back flow through the valve stops: the length of the murmur thus depends on the severity of the lesion and the compliance of the left ventricle. In severe cases, the murmur lasts throughout diastole and may be associated with gallop rhythm.

The inevitable increase in left ventricular stroke volume ordinarily cause a systolic murmur that is of no value in diagnosis or in the differentiation of aortic incompetence from predominant aortic stenosis. The site at which the immediate diastolic murmur of aortic incompetence is heard best depends on the degree of aortic dilatation. If the aorta is large, as in syphilitic lesions, the murmur is heard best to the right of the sternum. If the aorta is small, as in rheumatic lesions, the murmur is heard best to the left of the sternum. The murmur of aortic incompetence is sometimes only heard in the lower intercostal spaces (fourth or fifth) beside the sternum and is usually not heard well at the apex. When aortic incompetence is severe, an additional separate apical diastolic murmur is heard. This murmur, which is called an Austin Flint murmur, is mid-diastolic or presystolic and is thought to be due to fluttering of the anterior, aortic cusp of the mitral valve as it is caught between the two streams of blood flowing into the ventricle during diastole, one from the aorta and the other from the left atrium. Atrial contraction can influence the pattern of flow in this region and cause presystolic accentuation of the murmur, which is only heard in patients with severe aortic incompetence. Thus, the differential diagnosis is not between mitral stenosis and aortic incompetence, but between aortic incompetence and aortic incompetence plus mitral stenosis.

Although murmurs of aortic incompetence are similar in both the acute and the chronic form, the physical signs due to the hemodynamic effects of aortic incompetence may be strikingly different in the two lesions. For example, left ventricular dilatation and hypertrophy and aortic dilatation are not seen at the onset of acute aortic incompetence, whereas peripheral circulatory collapse, sweating, marked tachycardia, and signs of shock, with tachypnea, basal rales, and other signs of acute severe incompetence are not seen in patients with chronic lesions, except in severe left ventricular failure. The aortic diastolic murmur and the pulse pressure are the two sign that should be monitored continuously in patients with infective endocarditis who are at risk of developing aortic incompetence.

Differential Diagnosis

A. **Pulmonary Incompetence**: The murmur of aortic incompetence can be readily confused with the murmur of pulmonary incompetence in patients with severe pulmonary hypertension. Pulmonary incompetence rarely occurs in patients who do not have moderate or severe pulmonary hypertension. In patients with pulmonary hypertension, the hypertrophied right ventricle relaxes at about the same time as the left ventricle, causing the characteristic immediate, high-pitched diastolic murmur that is indistinguishable from that of aortic incompetence. On the basis of statistics, aortic incompetence is always the more likely lesion when an immediate diastolic murmur is present. However, full study is usually needed to confirm the

cause of the murmur, and the associated signs of pulmonary hypertension and right ventricular hypertrophy are ultimately always more important in diagnosis than the characteristics of the murmur.

In patients with low pulmonary arterial pressure, the murmur of pulmonary incompetence is different and is therefore not likely to be confused with an aortic murmur. When pulmonary arterial pressure is low, the right ventricle relaxes more slowly and the murmur starts later and is not a high-pitched.

B. **Rapid Aortic Runoff in other Conditions**: Disorder other than aortic incompetence can cause the characteristic physical signs of rapid runoff of blood from the aorta into some low-pressure area or into other areas in the circulation. These disorders include patent ductus arteriosus, aortopulmonary window, aortic-to-right-ventricular or atrial fistula, systemic arteriovenous fistula, truncus arteriosus, and associated ventricular septal defect. Anemia without organic valvular disease occasionally causes aortic incompetence.

MULTIPLE VALVE INVOLVEMENT

Combined Mitral and Aortic Valve Disease

Involvement of both aortic and mitral valves is almost pathognomonic of rheumatic heart disease, and patients with lesions of both valves have a higher incidence of infection in childhood (70%) than any other group of patients with valve disease. When both aortic and mitral valves are involved, the variability of the clinical picture greatly increases. The importance of the lesion at each valve can vary; the nature of each lesion (stenosis, incompetence, or mixture of the two) is diverse; and rheumatic myocardial involvement tends to play a more important part in the clinical course because the rheumatic infection is more severe and more often recurrent in these cases. It can be seen from the classification of mitral and aortic disease in this text that 20 or more sub-classifications of different mixed valvular diseases can be described. It is beyond the scope of this text to do more than point out some of the more obvious relationships between aortic and mitral disease and to make a few general comments about the clinical picture. Combined mitral and aortic valve disease constitutes about 10% of cases of valvular disease. Such patients have hemodynamically significant disease of each valve. Predominant aortic and predominant mitral diseases are about equal in frequency in combined lesions. Mitral stenosis decreases the apparent severity of aortic disease, particularly in aortic incompetence, and the combination of mitral stenosis and aortic incompetence is surprisingly well tolerated. After mitral stenosis has been relieved by valvotomy, aortic incompetence often appears to be more severe, and the presence on the ECG of left ventricular hypertrophy owing to aortic incompetence in a patient with predominant mitral stenosis is sufficient warning to warrant serious consideration of aortic valve replacement at the time of mitral valve surgery.

Mitral stenosis and aortic stenosis tend to mask one another, so that one or the other appears to be the dominant lesion clinically. The significance of the less dominant lesion is often underestimated.

When aortic valve disease is the major lesion, significant mitral incompetence is more serious that mitral stenosis. In either aortic stenosis or aortic incompetence, mitral incompetence is aggravated, and extreme cardiac enlargement and early heart failure are common.

Among the characteristic clinical pictures of combined valvular disease, which should be mentioned, is the combination of aortic stenosis with insignificant or mild mitral incompetence. This lesion gives rise to a characteristic high-pitched "seagull cry" murmur. In some cases, extension of aortic calcification into the aortic cusp of the mitral valve can be demonstrated, and this is one of the few combined aortic and mitral valve lesions that does not always have a rheumatic origin.

Clinical Course of Combined Lesions

Patients with combined mitral and aortic valve lesions tend to be symptomatic at an earlier age than patients with single valve lesions. The heart is usually larger, and atrial fibrillation tends to develop at an earlier age. The disease of each valve is less advanced in combined lesions because the valvular lesions are additive and because myocardial disease is so often present. Physical signs are more difficult to interpret in mixed lesions, and it is not always easy to distinguish the delayed diastolic or presystolic murmur of severe aortic incompetence (Austin Flint murmur) from the murmur of associated mitral stenosis. Similarly, an immediate basal diastolic murmur of pulmonary incompetence (Garham Steell murmur) in mitral stenosis with a raised pulmonary vascular resistance can be confused with the murmur of associated aortic incompetence. In patients with predominant aortic valve disease, the distinction between functional and organic mitral incompetence is often difficult. In the presence of left heart failure, a systolic murmur of mitral incompetence is often found, but it may be difficult to distinguish from the aortic systolic murmur. In mixed mitral stenosis and incompetence, the organic nature of the systolic murmur can be more readily recognized. In combined aortic and mitral valve disease, either valve lesion may become acutely worse in the course of infective endocarditis. The presence of a chronic lesion of one valve exaggerates the effects of an acute lesion of the other valve. Infective endocarditis and systemic embolism are as common in combined aortic and mitral valve disease as they are in aortic or mitral incompetence alone.

Combined Mitral and Tricuspid Valve Disease

Functional tricuspid incompetence has already been mentioned as a common complication of mitral stenosis with raised pulmonary vascular resistance. In about 2% of patients with mitral valve disease, organic tricuspid valve disease is present and causes right heart failure. The mitral valve lesion is usually mixed mitral stenosis and incompetence, and pulmonary vascular resistance is not greatly raised (average 2 mm Hg/L/min). Markedly raised systemic venous pressure (average 24 mm Hg) is the most striking clinical feature, and cardiac enlargement is usually massive, but not as great as in giant left atrium. Low cardiac output and atrial fibrillation are almost inevitable, and the lesions tend to run a chronic course in which valve replacement provides less benefit than in disease of the mitral valve alone. Isolated tricuspid valve disease without mitral valve involvement can theoretically occur, but for practical purposes, it is rare enough to be of negligible importance.

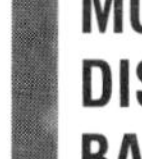

MODIFIED VALVULAR HEART DISEASE SECONDARY TO SURGERY/ BALLOON MITRAL VALVOTOMY

Mitral Valvotomy

Mitral commissurotomy is the most important iatrogenic factor modifying the course of valvular heart disease. Tight mitral stenosis and mitral stenosis with raised pulmonary vascular resistance were usually fatal in early middle life before the advent of mitral valve surgery. Even relatively ineffective closed mitral valvotomy was—and still is—capable of influencing the clinical course of mitral stenosis. The operation is palliative rather than curative, and in 2–15 years after valvotomy, the patient is likely to experience a recurrence of dyspnea. In some cases (about 20%), a second valvotomy is performed, but in most cases, mitral valve replacement is necessary at the second operation. The clinical features of these patients with iatrogenically modified mitral stenosis warrant description.

Clinical Findings

Symptoms

In patients who have had a previous mitral valvotomy, symptoms are difficult to assess.

Dyspnea is the commonest symptom, and, as in all patients with mitral valve disease, the relation between the onset of atrial fibrillation and the onset of dyspnea is of prime importance. A clinical picture resembling that of mixed mitral valve disease is common. Patients who have gained relief through mitral valvotomy are likely to experience a significant increase in dyspnea when atrial fibrillation occurs at about age 40. There is often a relationship between the length of the asymptomatic interval following valvotomy and the age of the patient. A woman who has had a mitral valvotomy in her 20s is likely to have 15 symptom-free years old woman is likely to develop atrial fibrillation within about 5 years of operation. It seems that mitral valvotomy is a means of shifting the patient from the category of pure tight mitral stenosis to that of mixed mitral stenosis and incompetence.

Signs

The physical signs in iatrogenically modified cases usually reflect the preoperative findings. A loud opening snap and loud first heart sound are often present, and the timing of the opening snap reflects the preoperative and not the postoperative status of the patient. In such cases, the length of the diastolic murmur measured at the bedside becomes the best indicator of the severity of stenosis. A systolic murmur may appear after surgery, but, as is the case in patients who have not undergone operation, its significance is open to discussion.

Electrocardiographic Findings

In a few cases, regression of the changes of right ventricular hypertrophy are seen, but in most patients the ECG shows little change from the preoperative tracing. Eventually, atrial fibrillation will almost certainly develop.

X-Ray Findings

The absence of the left atrial appendage as a bulge on the left heart border is a characteristic finding in patients who have undergone operation. If the pulmonary artery was enlarged before operation, it seldom returns to normal size, and the same is true of the left atrium. Changes in the degree of pulmonary congestions are perhaps the best indicators of the success of surgical treatment.

PATIENTS WITH ARTIFICIAL VALVES

Some patients visit doctor after corrective surgery, patients who have had mitral or aortic valve replacement are becoming more common in everyday medical practice. By far the largest number of such patients have Starr-Edwards ball and cage prostheses. Other forms of plastic and metal valves, such as the Bjork-Shiley disk valve, and homograft or heterograft (Hancock) tissue valves are also used.

The clinical picture in patients who have had valve replacement varies greatly and depends on the type of valve used, the nature of the original lesion, the stage at which operation was performed, and the success of the operation. Few patients are free of symptoms; the problems encountered are most commonly related to thrombosis, embolism, leakage or obstruction of the valve, and hemorrhage from excessive anticoagulant therapy.

Clinical Findings

Symptoms

Many patients with artificial valves have residual shortness of breath on exertion. Most have at least a small pressure gradient across the valve at rest that becomes larger when the cardiac output and heart rate increase during exercise. The patient may also complain of the loud noise made by the artificial valve as it opens and closes with each heartbeat, but most patients become accustomed to the sensation within a few weeks after operation.

Signs

The physical signs arising from an artificial valve depend on the nature and type of valve used. Tissue valves do not give rise to the loud opening and closing clicks heard with metal and plastics prostheses. However, they do tend to leak with the passage of time as the tissue stiffens and calcified. Thus, mitral systolic and aortic diastolic murmurs are not uncommon. The opening and closing clicks of plastic and metal valves are characteristic for each individual brand of valve. In general, there is a loud opening click at the start of systole and a loud closing click at the end of systole. The clicks are usually louder than the normal heart sounds and interfere with auscultation of natural valves. Systolic and diastolic murmurs are difficult to interpret in patients with artificial valves, and more importance should be given to changes in the auscultatory findings than to the findings themselves.

Signs of pulmonary congestion and right heart failure with edema and a raised venous pressure are found when surgical results are poor.

Differential Diagnosis

The principal problem in differential diagnosis is distinguishing artificial valve malfunction from disease of another valve. Full study of the patients is needed in such cases, and the findings vary greatly in individual patients. Color Doppler is very useful.

Complications

Thrombosis around the artificial valve, with consequent stenosis and systemic embolism, is the commonest complication of artificial valves. Anticoagulant therapy is needed in all types of valves except tissue valves, and hemorrhage due to excessive anticoagulation is also encountered. When thrombus forms around a prosthetic valve, it may disturb valve function and interfere with both the opening and the closing of the valve. Thus, both stenosis and incompetence can result from thrombus formation around an artificial valve. In some cases, especially early after operation, valve displacement due to tearing out of the sutures anchoring the valve leads to paravalvular leak. In other cases, the valve mechanism itself may fail and cause leakage. Sudden death is still an important complication of valve replacement. The mechanism is not always clear, but escape of a worn ball from the cage mechanism sticks shut. Hemolysis may occur after valve replacement. Mechanical trauma to the red cells resulting from contact with the artificial valve is thought to be responsible. Infective endocarditis can also occur when the endothelialized surface of the prosthetic valve becomes infected. Infection at this site is particularly difficult to eradicate, and removal of the infected prosthesis and replacement are often necessary.

Chapter **5**

Infective Endocarditis

▎ CHANGING CHARACTERISTICS OF ENDOCARDITIS

Use of the term infective endocarditis reflects the view that it is no longer appropriate to think of acute and subacute endocarditis as separate diseases or to think only of bacteria as possible causes. Endocarditis now appears in so many forms and is caused by so many different organisms, bacterial and fungal, that the classic distinction between acute and subacute forms has become blurred and artificial. Some cases are hyperacute, some are chronic, and the range of severity frustrates any attempt at neat classification into two types. The same organism may cause either acute or subacute endocarditis depending on its virulence and the status of the host defenses.

The clinical features of infective endocarditis have changed to some degree as a result of factors that play a role both in producing the disease and in modifying its course. While classic cases of subacute bacterial endocarditis due to *Streptococcus viridans* in chronic rheumatically diseased valves still occur, new forms of the disease are seen in which infection occurs in a patient who is already taking one or more antibiotics on a long- or short-term basis. Such patients may have subacute infections with virulent organisms or low-grade infections with exotic organisms not ordinarily encountered in "spontaneously" occurring disease.

Changing Etiology and Symptoms

Many of the classic features of subacute bacterial endocarditis that occurred commonly before the antibiotic era are less frequent now because of antibiotic therapy, which is commonly used for any symptoms resembling "flu". Such treatment suppresses but usually does not eradicate the bloodstream infection. As a result, a new "iatrogenecally subacute" form of endocarditis is seen, with an altered pattern of causative organisms. In the past, *S. viridans* was responsible for 90–95% of cases of subacute bacterial endocarditis, but this organism is now responsible for only about half of cases and about one-third of all cases of infective endocarditis. The relative frequency of infections with *Staphylococcus faecalis* (enterococcus), gram-negative organisms both aerobic and anaerobic, yeasts, and molds are increasing at the expense of *S. viridans*. Each of these organisms may cause either acute or subacute endocarditis. Infections with certain organisms (e.g. *Bacteroides*) are still infrequent, but all rare organisms must now be considered possible causative agents.

Special Valve and Congenital Factors

Tricuspid lesions are involved in infective endocarditis almost exclusively in intravenous drug users, and the relative frequency of left and right sided lesions in such patients varies in different cities and institutions. Pulmonary stenosis, patent ductus arteriosus, ventricular septal defect, and bicuspid aortic valve are the most common congenital cardiac lesions in which endocarditis develop. Infective endocarditis is rare in atrial septal defect.

Precipitating Factors

A precipitating factor should always be sought. Dental procedures, recent instrumentation of the genitourinary tract, gynecologic procedures, or inflammatory gastrointestinal disease sometimes precedes the illness. In about half of subacute cases, no cause can be established; fewer cases of acute endocarditis are of unknown cause. In acute infective endocarditis, septicemia due to any cause, plus the special situation previously mentioned, is often present.

Other Factors and Influences

Embolism from discharge of fragments of the vegetation into the systemic or pulmonary circulation is responsible for many of the clinical features, as will be noted later. Surgical drainage in addition to antibiotics may be required for metastatic abscesses.

Endocarditis is more apt to occur in patients with mild to moderate valvular disease. For example, it is rare in severe mitral stenosis and infrequent in patients with established atrial fibrillation.

Host defenses with antibody formation, local attempts at repair, and local macrophage infiltration can be seen at autopsy but rarely are adequate in them to clear the infection. Age is a factor; most cases occur in young adults, but older and younger persons are not immune to the disease. At present, the age distribution is bimodal, with younger individuals most apt to have acute infective endocarditis and older ones subacute endocarditis, probably because of the presence of unoperated rheumatic valvular disease in the older patients. Current data indicate that the median age at onset is 45 years, that 25% of patients are over 60 years of age, and that only 7% are under 20 years of age.

Subacute Infective Endocarditis

Diagnosis (Fig. 5.1)

The onset of endocarditis may be chronic and insidious, and unless one searches for infections due to bacteria or fungi in every patient in whom the combination of fever and valvular lesions coexists, the diagnosis can be missed for weeks or months. The presenting symptoms are usually nonspecific and are often attributed to a febrile illness because the symptoms include fever, malaise, arthralgia, muscle pains with fatigue, and chills with high fever in the acute varieties. if short-term antibiotic treatment is given, the clinical picture is that of recurrent "flu".

The diagnostic features of endocarditis can be categorized under the headings fever and infection, valvular lesions, and evidence of systemic or pulmonary emboli. If the diagnosis is suspected from the presence of a murmur or valve lesion, fever, and emboli, blood cultures must be obtained.

A. **Fever:** Fever is the most frequent presenting sign and may appear without apparent predisposing cause or may follow a major or minor surgical procedure. Prostatic and other urogenital operations in men and dilatation and curettage of the uterus, septic abortion, and other gynecologic procedures in women are sometimes precursors of endocarditis, both acute and subacute. Weakness, malaise, and loss of weight without fever may occur in debilitated or elderly patients, especially if antibiotics have been given even in small doses, and may occasionally be due to acute renal failure secondary to endocarditis. The symptoms may be overlooked in elderly patients, in whom the diagnosis is often missed or is made only at autopsy. The higher mortality rate in these patients is probably due to delayed diagnosis and thus delayed onset of effective antibiotic therapy. In uremic, elderly, and debilitated patients, fever is often absent.

B. **Emboli:** Acute systemic embolism may be the presenting symptom and may occur at

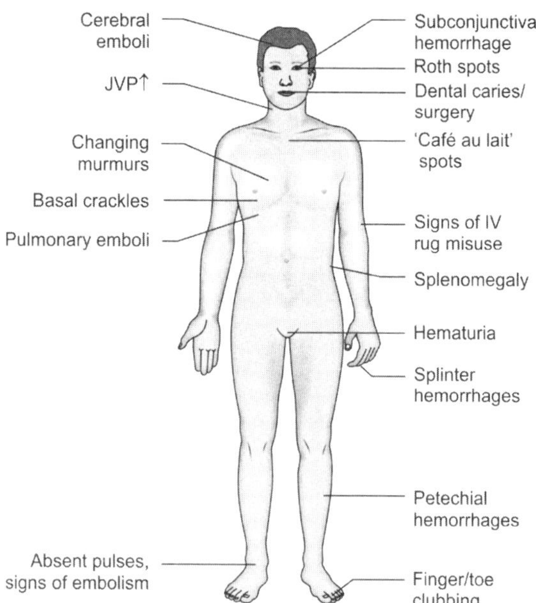

Fig. 5.1: Clinical features of endocarditis

any time during the course of the disease. Emboli are usually small except in *Candida* or *Serratia* infections (acute or chronic) and are usually characterized by microscopic hematuria (which may also be due to immune complex disease) or petechiae. Osler's nodes, one of the best-known manifestations of infective endocarditis, were described by Osler in 1893 as ephemeral, painful, nodular erythematous spots on the skin, chiefly of the hands and feet. The site where the lesions eventually appear is usually painful first. Although Osler thought that these cutaneous manifestations were probably caused by minute emboli, other investigators have thought that they might be due to an immune mechanism. However, aspirates from the nodes both during life and at autopsy reveal pathogenic organisms, and histologic examination reveals a microabscess in the papillary dermis, together with microemboli in the nearby dermal arterioles, making suspect the theory of vasculitis resulting from an immunologic reaction. Nontender nodules on the soles of the feet and the palms of the hands (Janeway's lesion) are thought now to be a hypersensitivity reaction or deposit of immune complex but were formerly thought to be emboli. Emboli to the systemic circulation are uncommon in right sided valvular lesions of acute endocarditis; the right sided manifestations are recurrent pneumonia or pulmonary embolism. *Jockman's dictum:* If a person with valvular defect but without atrial fibrillation develops systemic embolism—suspect infective endocarditis.

1. **Small emboli:** In left-sided lesions, emboli to the skin may be manifested by splinter hemorrhages in the nails of the fingers or toes (but these may occur in individuals engaged in manual labor). Petechiae (usually on the conjunctiva or hard palate or around the neck and upper trunk) are more definite evidence of embolism. At first, they are red and small, but when observed over a period of days they become brown and gradually fade. Hemorrhagic areas with white centers may be seen in the fundi owing to emboli in the nerve fiber retinal layer (Roth spots). These are

less common than petechiae. Emboli to the kidney may cause flank pain or microscopic hematuria. Petechiae and microscopic hematuria must be sought every day.

2. **Large emboli**: Large emboli may involve, (1) the cerebral arteries, causing hemiplegia, other central nervous system deficit, neurologic syndromes including headache, psychiatric symptoms, confusion, or sterile meningitis; (2) the coronary arteries, resulting in acute myocardial infarction: or (3) the vasa vasorum, leading to mycotic aneurysms. These last may rupture, often after prodromal symptoms of headache and somnolence, if they involve the cerebral arteries. When such prodromal symptoms are present, cerebral angiography should be performed to establish the presence of mycotic aneurysms so that appropriate surgical therapy can be planned. Mycotic aneurysms may appear anywhere, often in branches of the renal artery. Rupture is infrequent, and these lesions are often missed.

3. **Septic abscesses**: If staphylococci are the infecting organisms in either acute or subacute cases, septic abscesses may develop, especially in the liver, kidney, brain and spleen and treatment will be unavailing until the lesion is drained surgically. Septic abscesses may contribute to continued fever and require surgical incision even though the organisms on the endocardium of the valves have been eradicated.

4. **Splenomegaly and clubbed fingers**: These are less common in acute endocarditis and in subacute cases of short duration. They are usually late signs in untreated patients and, although they were common in the preantibiotic era, are much less common today (approximately 10% of cases). As in any systemic infection, splenomegaly may occur, although it is less frequent when antibiotic therapy is given early in the course of the disease.

C. **Immune Complex Nephritis and Renal Emboli**: Glomerulonephritis and renal failure are frequently seen in infective endocarditis and were formerly thought to be embolic in origin. More recently, it has become evident that the renal lesions are immunologic in origin and are due to the deposit of antigen antibody complexes and complement on the glomerular basement membrane. Immunofluorescence of renal biopsy specimens demonstrates granular deposits of 1gM and C3 in all glomeruli studies. The antigen in glomerular deposits corresponds to the organism found in blood cultures.

D. **Anemia**: Normocytic anemia is common, especially in long-standing infection, and probably accounts in part for the weakness and lassitude seen in patients with chronic infective endocarditis.

E. **Cardiac Findings:** Symptoms of heart disease such as dyspnea or palpitations develop late in subacute (in contract to acute) infective endocarditis, and the cardiac origin of the illness may only be suspected if a known valvular lesion or murmurs are present or if embolic manifestations appear.

In subacute infective endocarditis, a murmur is almost always present, indicating previous valve involvement of rheumatic or congenital origin. The valve involvement is usually mild to moderate, and patients may not know they have a cardiac lesion. Careful auscultation for the presence of such a lesion is mandatory in suspicious cases, and subacute endocarditis is an important cause of fever of unknown origin in patients in whom cardiac disease is overlooked.

Recently, it has been appreciated that lesions heretofore not considered to be possible predisposing causes of subacute infective endocarditis may in fact be important etiologic factors. These included prolapsed mitral valve (systolic click-murmur syndrome), fibrosis and calcification of the annulus of the mitral valve, and atherosclerosis of the aortic ring and valve. Prolapse of the mitral valve can often be demonstrated by echocardiography or angiography. Echocardiography may also be helpful and occasionally is diagnostic in doubtful cases of vegetations on the aortic valve, especially if they are large (> 5 mm), as in fungal infections. Echocardiography is less helpful when endocarditis involves the mitral valve.

Changing murmurs help in diagnosis of acute infective endocarditis when the fulminant valve lesions progress rapidly. They are much less helpful in subacute infective endocarditis, when the changing murmurs are probably due in large part to anemia, tachycardia or other hemodynamic variables that change from one time of examination to another. The abrupt appearance of a diastolic murmur, such as that of aortic insufficiently, is more helpful, as are the developing signs of tricuspid insufficiency in acute infective endocarditis.

Cardiac failure formerly was a late occurrence, as was the development of atrial fibrillation. Untreated patients often died of infection before cardiac failure could develop. Early cardiac failure is frequent today in acute cases, but in subacute cases, it may not occur until months after bacteriologic cure, as infection heals and valve lesions worsen (especially aortic valve lesions). Pericarditis is infrequent.

Acute Infective Endocarditis

The circumstances in which acute infective endocarditis occurs are discussed above. This section will emphasize the differences between acute and subacute endocarditis but will discuss also the organisms, the involved valve, and the hemodynamic effects.

Diagnosis

The infection is apt to be more abrupt, with higher fever, chills, and the presence of septic abscesses because the predominant organism is usually *S. aureus*, even in heroin addicts who infect the mixture injected with organisms already present in the nose, throat, and skin. In California, *Candida parapsilosis* and *Serratia marcescens* were unusually frequent organisms. The symptoms of infection usually predominate, and organisms are more easily cultured and identified than in subacute cases. When the lesion is on the tricuspid valve, however, pulmonary complications of pneumonia, pulmonary embolism, and pulmonary abscess are dominant. X-rays of the chest reveal pleural effusions and changing pulmonary infiltrates of variable size and shape that may recur. The same is true of subacute right-sided lesions, which are rare. Splenomegaly and clubbed fingers are less frequent. The major postmortem lesions in patients with *S aureus* endocarditis are listed.

A. **Emboli:** In fungal endocarditis, emboli are more frequent and can be large and disabling. Cerebral embolism may produce hemiplegia, and the possibility of endocarditis must always be considered in patients who develop acute stroke. Smaller emboli, such as petechiae, are less frequent than in subacute bacterial endocarditis, and the same is true of splinter hemorrhages and Osler's nodes. The decreased frequency of systemic embolism in acute infective endocarditis is due to the frequency of right-sided lesions as well as to the rapid downhill course resulting from the server infection.

B. **Cardiac Findings:**

1. **Changing murmurs and valve findings**: The frequency with which acute infective endocarditis occurs on normal cardiac valves makes serial examination more important than is the case in subacute endocarditis. The development of murmurs and evidence of valvular involvement may be noted if the patient is under close observation as the infection on the valve increases and the vegetations become larger. This is especially true of tricuspid insufficiency in heroin addicts, and careful examination may disclose the progressive appearance and lengthening of a tricuspid systolic murmur, made

worse by inspiration as right atrial inflow increases with inspiration. A right-sided gallop rhythm may appear, as may the progressive development of a prominent v wave in the jugular venous pulse and enlargement of a tender, pulsating liver, with right-sided failure. Valvular vegetations can be demonstrated by echocardiography. When acute infective endocarditis, involves the aortic valve, the diastolic murmur may be long and soft and the first sound may be soft because of early closure of the mitral valve. The diastolic pressure may be maintained by reflex peripheral arteriolar vasoconstriction, and early mitral valve closure may be a sign of increasing aortic insufficiency. As the magnitude of the aortic regurgitant flow increases, there is a rapid early diastolic rise in left ventricular pressure and left atrial pressure before the onset of systole, causing a prominent Austin Flint diastolic murmur. These findings are not specific for endocarditis. If hemodynamic measurements are made, the crossover of left ventricular enddiastolic pressure and left atrial pressure precedes the Q wave of the ECG instead of slightly following it at the peak or down stroke of the R wave. Early closure of the mitral valve can be clearly demonstrated on echocardiography, when the anterior and posterior leaflets approximate each other well before the onset of the Q wave of the ECG with a normal P-R interval. This ominous sign is a harbinger of severe left ventricular failure. The magnitude of the acute aortic insufficiency can also be shown by supra-aortic cineangiography, which shows the left ventricle fully opacified in a single beat of the regurgitant flow.

2. **Cardiac failure**: Cardiac failure is the most feared complication of acute infective endocarditis and may occur with startling rapidity in left-sided lesions, whether mitral or aortic. One cannot use the width of the pulse pressure, the loudness of the murmur, or the size of the left ventricle as a guide to the severity or imminence of left ventricular failure. The left ventricle is often only slightly enlarged, and the ECG may not reveal left ventricular hypertrophy in acute as compared to chronic aortic insufficiency because of the rapid development of aortic or mitral insufficiency. Symptoms of pulmonary edema and echocardiographic evidence of marked early closure of a mitral valve lead the physician to suspect perforation or destruction of the aortic valve and indicate the need for valve replacement. Vigorous medical treatment may be needed while the infection subsides so that the sutures will hold. Careful judgment is required to determine the timing of operation if cardiac failure worsens despite control of the infection.

3. **Ventricular septum and muscle involvement**: The infection on the aortic valve may spread to the ventricular septum, and abscesses may develop and rupture into the right heart or may interfere with conduction of the cardiac impulse and cause atrioventricular block with or without syncope. Septic abscesses can be suspected, if there is sudden development of atrioventricular block or hemiblock. Mitral valve infections may cause septic abscesses of the papillary muscles or destruction of the mitral ring, resulting in flail mitral valves that require prompt surgical correction.

Differential Diagnosis

Infective endocarditis must be differentiated from all other causes of prolonged and obscure fever. The diagnosis is based on a positive blood culture in conjunction with the presence of a valve lesion and the absence of diagnostic signs or tests supporting an alternative diagnosis. Infection, neoplasm, and connective tissue disorders are the most common causes of fever of unknown origin (40%, 20% and 20% respectively), and these must be excluded.

The major difficulty in diagnosis occurs when blood cultures are negative, which means that reliance must be placed on associated diagnostic features. This emphasizes the importance of optimally obtained and examined blood cultures.

1. Bacteremia may be due to pneumonia, septic thrombophlebitis, meningitis, cellulitis, or infected fistulas. There must be evidence of valve lesions as well as emboli before septicemia can be considered to have originated in the heart. Miliary tuberculosis must be kept in mind and serial chest X-rays obtained.

2. Acute rheumatic fever occasionally is confusing, but only if blood cultures are negative. In acute rheumatic fever, the arthralgia or arthritis responds rapidly to salicylates, and there may be erythema marginatum, chorea, or previous beta-streptococcal infection which can be documented by increasing antistreptolysin O titers in the serum.

3. Neoplasm can be diagnosed by appropriate measures or by biopsy of lymph nodes or bone marrow. If atrial myxoma is suspected, echocardiography and angiography can be diagnostic.

4. Connective tissue disorders must be suspected and diagnosed on the basis of skin or renal lesions, a positive LE cell preparation or antinuclear antibody test, renal biopsy, and negative blood cultures.

Prosthetic Valve Endocarditis

Endocarditis on a prosthetic valve occurs in 1–4% of patients and is one of the most disturbing postoperative complications of prosthetic valve surgery. Most cases have involved the aortic valve, but the mitral valve may be infected as well. Infection may occur early, within a month or 2 of surgery, or late, as with any diseased valve. The early onset of infection is thought to be caused by organisms introduced at the time of surgery from such sources as an infected pump oxygenator, contaminated intravenous lines used during the procedure, or infected personnel. A postoperative wound infection, especially of the sternum, may be a source of infection of the prosthetic valve. Although only one-third of infections of prosthetic valves occur early (within the first 2 months), the mortality rate is high (70–80%) in the early-onset cases as compared to the more frequent late-onset endocarditis (often many months to a year or so after the valve was introduced). The late-onset cases have a lower mortality rate; the overall mortality rate of all cases of prosthetic valve endocarditis approximates 50–60%. The causes of early death in Wilson's 1975 series were prosthetic valve dysfunction, infection, cardiac failure, and emboli.

Early-onset endocarditis of a prosthetic valve is usually due to *S. aureus* or a gram-negative organism, whereas late-onset endocarditis is usually due to *S. viridans* or to gram-negative bacilli. *Candida* infections are most apt to occur early rather than late.

Late-onset endocarditis usually follows one of the common predisposing causes of endocarditis on a damaged valve and pathologically involves the neoendothelium, which grows over cloth-covered valves.

It is of interest that on pathologic examination, all patients with prosthetic valve endocarditis have infection located behind the site of attachment of the prosthesis to the valve ring, with spread to the neighboring structures. Severe regurgitation through the involved valve follows the prosthetic detachment and may require urgent surgery.

Chapter 6

Myocardial Disease

■ INTRODUCTION

Myocarditis and Cardiomyopathy

This chapter discusses myocarditis, cardiomyopathy, and various diseases and clinical states of which disease of the myocardium may be a manifestation. It deals with hypertrophic cardiomyopathy (often called idiopathic hypertrophic subaortic stenosis, or IHSS) under a separate heading because the overall clinical picture and mode of presentation of the patient with hypertrophic cardiomyopathy, with murmurs suggestive of valvular disease, lead the physician to an entirely different set of investigative procedures from those indicated in the management of patients with idiopathic cardiomyopathy, in whom systemic and pulmonary congestion are the principal features.

The common known causes of chronic myocardial disease (ischemic, hypertensive, valvular, congenital, as well as infective endocarditis and syphilis) are also to be considered.

General Considerations

Diseases of the myocardium form a complex and heterogeneous group of diseases that are somewhat confusing chiefly because they are due to varied causes, not all of them known, but also because the clinical manifestations vary from a trivial illness recognized only by non-specific electrocardiographic abnormalities, mild chest pain, or slight enlargement of the heart to fulminant cardiac failure with severe dyspnea, gallop rhythm, hypotension, tachycardia, recurrent ventricular arrhythmias, and death, which may occur suddenly and unexpectedly. Myocarditis may be acute or chronic, and the acute form may be benign or fulminant. The terms chronic myocarditis and chronic cardiomyopathy are often used interchangeably, since the cause is often unknown and because the inflammatory infiltrate suggests infection ("-itis"). "Chronic idiopathic cardiomyopathy" goes by a variety of names, none of them entirely satisfactory, including Fiedler's myocarditis, idiopathic myocarditis, primary myocardial, disease, "vexation of the heart", endocardial myofibrosis, Loeffler's syndrome and alcoholic cardiomyopathy. Myocarditis may be primary in the heart, or the myocardial disease may be secondary to systemic diseases such as the connective tissue disorders.

Some forms of myocardial disease are much more common in tropical and subtropical areas than in temperate climates. The reasons for this geographic distribution are not definitely known, but nutritional factors are thought to be responsible. The diagnosis is often made by exclusion, especially in the case of idiopathic cardiomyopathy, and the physician must consider common diseases in the differential diagnosis that may have unusual clinical features such as ischemic cardiomyopathy, "burned-out" hypertension, rheumatic heart disease, and congenital heart disease. Cardiomyopathy is apparently increasing in frequency for reasons that are totally obscure; as congenital and rheumatic heart disease in adults become less common, cardiomyopathy and the acute myocarditis have come to form a larger percentage of cases of cardiac disease.

Myocarditis is often associated with pericarditis, especially in viral infections. The endocardium and the valves are less often involved except in the case of acute rheumatic fever or endocardial fibrosis. Myocardial disease due to drug toxicity is becoming increasingly common with use of cardiotoxic drugs such as the phenothiazines, doxorubicin, the corticosteroids, emetine, and antimony as well as those that may cause lupus erythematosus, e.g. procainamide, hydralazine, and phenytoin.

Non-viral myocarditis is recognized on the basis of the obvious manifestations of the underlying disease, as in diphtheria, rheumatic fever, or pneumococcal pneumonia. Chagas disease is endemic in South and Central America but rare in the USA, and the diagnosis of acute myocarditis is usually based on epidemiologic evidence as well as the presence of a chagoma at the site of entry of the parasites and recovery of trypanosomes in blood drawn early in the course of the disease. If the patient lives in a thatched hut in which the *Triatoma* vector lives, the diagnosis should be considered.

Acute rheumatic fever is associated with other major findings such as arthritis and a history of recent streptococcal infection. Arthritis is relieved by salicylates, and recent streptococcal infection can be inferred from finding increasing titers of antistreptolysin antibodies in the serum. Diphtheria causes a typical lesion in the throat but may infect the skin also, and the organism can be identified from throat and skin cultures. In acute myocardial toxicity from drugs, awareness of the use of drugs, their dosage, and the presence of the disease being treated with drugs helps to differentiate myocardial toxicity from acute myocarditis. This may be quite difficult in patients with acute lupus erythematosus with fever, pericarditis, and vasculitis, and specific diagnostic procedures

such as lupus erythematosus preparations and serial neutralizing antibody determinations for vital infections may be required to make the determination.

Acute glomerulonephritis may present as acute cardiac failure, but the poststreptococcal state, hypertension, and urinary findings should make the diagnosis clear. Hemodynamic findings indicate that "cardiac failure" in acute nephritis is usually due to salt and water retention and not to cardiac failure per se. The cardiac index is often increased, averaging 5.4 liters/min/m^2 at rest and 7.54 liters/min/m^2 with exercise in contrast to the low cardiac output in acute cardiac failure. The pulmonary capillary wedge pressure is slightly increased at rest but within the normal range after exercise (averaging 15 mm Hg at rest and 18 mm Hg after exercise).

■ RHEUMATIC FEVER

All undergraduate and postgraduate students must be expert in rheumatic fever. Rheumatic fever is a subacute or chronic systemic disease, which for unknown reasons may either be self-limiting or lead to slowly progressive valvular deformity. Rarely, it is acute and fulminant. It is a much less common disease now, probably because of effective treatment of beta-hemolytic streptococcal infections, but it is still not uncommon.

Rheumatic fever and its sequelae used to be the commonest cause of heart disease in people under 50 years of age in the USA, and as a cause of heart disease in people of all ages, it ranked third behind hypertension and atherosclerotic coronary disease. The prevalence is probably much less now in developed countries, but the disease is still common elsewhere. Chorea is seen more frequently in females. The peak incidence occurs between the ages of 5 and 15; rheumatic fever is rare before age 4 and after age 50.

Etiology

Rheumatic fever is initiated by an infection with group A beta-hemolytic streptococci, appearing usually 1–4 weeks after an episode of tonsillitis, nasopharyngitis, or otitis media. The streptococcal infection is the antigen for the antigen-antibody response resulting in rheumatic fever. This nonpurulent complication of streptococcal infections should be differentiated from purulent complications such as peritonsillar abscess, sinusitis, mastoiditis, and cervical adenitis, among others that are so common in children.

Diagnosis

The diagnosis is more readily made in epidemics of streptococcal infections, which occur in wartime, when the relationship of β-hemolytic streptococcal infections and the subsequent nonsuppurative complications of rheumatic fever are more readily seen. Even mild cases can be recognized under these circumstances. When isolated cases of rheumatic fever occur, the diagnosis is often unsuspected and not made. This may explain the high percentage of patients with rheumatic heart disease who deny a previous history of rheumatic fever.

Children usually have a more fulminant disease than adults, and the diagnosis is therefore more easily made. In adults, the diagnosis is infrequently made except in "epidemics". The disease "licks the joints and bites the heart" of children, but the reverse is usually true of adults.

The diagnosis may be difficult, with scarcely diagnosable illness or it may be obvious, with all the criteria necessary for diagnosis. Because of the difficulties in interpreting the symptoms, the diagnostic findings have been separated into major and minor criteria, with at least two major criteria being necessary for diagnosis. The *major criteria* are peri-, myo-, endocarditis, chorea, subcutaneous nodules, erythema marginatum and polyarthritis. The *minor criteria* are fever, malaise, abdominal pain "growing pains", and laboratory findings of leukocytosis, raised sedimentation rate, and evidence of a preceding streptococcal infection (increased liter of antistreptolysin O), increased P-R on ECG.

Clinical Findings

Symptoms

The disease usually begins with either fever or arthritis in a patient who has recovered from a β-hemolytic streptococcal infection 2–3 weeks previously.

1. **Fever:** The fever may be low-grade and intermittent, but in severe cases with pericarditis or myocarditis, it may be substantial. It is a minor criterion of rheumatic fever because it may be due to many causes. The fever often lasts for weeks or months, in conjunction with general symptoms of malaise, asthenia, weight loss, and anorexia, which may indicate a smoldering rheumatic state but are also characteristic of any chronic active disease.

2. **Joint pains:** Growing pain in joints, periarticular tissues, or muscle systems may be a symptom of rheumatic fever but are not specific.

3. **Arthritis:** Arthritis with effusion is characteristically a migratory polyarthritis of gradual or sudden onset, which involves the large joints sequentially, one becoming hot, red, swollen, and tender as the inflammation in the previously involved joint subsides. Body temperature rises as each successive joint becomes inflamed. In adults, only a single joint may be affected. The acute arthritis lasts 1-5 weeks and subsides without residual deformity. Prompt response of arthritis to therapeutic doses of salicylates is characteristic of rheumatic fever.

4. **Peri: Myo-, Endocarditis:** The symptoms of carditis in rheumatic fever are often slight and must be looked for specifically. The patient does not complain of dyspnea unless cardiac failure is present. Chest pain is usually prominent, either made worse with breathing, related to posture if pericardial or epigastric if there is peritoneal involvement. The interpretation of the symptoms is clarified by signs, an ECG and X-ray findings. The patients may complain of palpitations due to a rapid heart rate, but symptoms of arrhythmia are uncommon.

5. **Skin lesions and subcutaneous nodules:** The patient may complain of skin lesions or subcutaneous nodules, but these are more frequently found on physical examination.

6. **Chorea:** Chorea consists of purposeless jerky movements, continual and non-repetitive, of the limbs, trunk, and facial muscles. Milder forms masquerade as undue restlessness as the patient attempts to convert uncontrolled movements into seemingly purposeful ones. Facial grimaces of infinite variety are common. These movements are made worse by emotional tension and disappear entirely during sleep. The episode lasts several weeks or occasionally months.

   Chorea may appear suddenly as an isolated entity with no 'minor criteria' or may develop in the course of overt rheumatic fever. Eventually, 50% of patients have other signs of rheumatic fever. Girls are more frequently affected, and occurrence in adults is rare.

Signs

1. **General appearance:** The patient may seem well or may appear both acutely and chronically ill, with pallor, subdued affect, and general debility.

2. **Arthritis:** The joint may be normal on examination in patients with arthralgia and growing pains, or reddened and swollen in acute arthritis. Movement of the involved joint or even the weight or movement of bed sheets over the joint is poorly tolerated. The arthritis may involve only one joint or may 'migrate' to involve multiple joints as the patient is examined daily. Often the initial joint improves as a new joint is affected, but occasionally polyarthritis is present.

3. **Carditis:** The myocardial signs may be minimal or characterized by tachycardia which is out of proportion to the fever and which persists during sleep and is greatly increased by slight activity; by cardiac enlargement with the cardiac impulse displaced to the left; by pericardial friction rub with or without a raised jugular venous pressure, depending on the presence and amount of pericardial effusion; by painful engorgement of the liver; and by signs of left ventricular failure such as gallop rhythm or pulmonary rales. Cardiac murmurs are infrequent at onset, but with the passage of days, careful auscultation may reveal a short, soft mid-diastolic murmur valve involvement, a short early diastolic murmur of aortic valve involvement, or a soft pansystolic murmur of mitral incompetence, which becomes louder during the course of the disease and is transmitted to the axilla. Short systolic murmur are common but are due to fever or tachycardia and not to mitral incompetence. The heart sounds may be 'tictac' as described in the section on acute myocarditis, and may change in quality on daily examination.

4. **Arrhythmias:** Premature beats may occur but are uncommon; atrial fibrillation and ventricular tachycardia are rare.

5. **Erythema marginatum (annulare):** This is frequently associated with skin nodules. The lesions begin as rapidly enlarging macules, which assume the shape of rings or crescents with clear centers. They may be slightly raised and confluent. The rash may be transient or may persist for long periods.

6. **Subcutaneous nodules:** These are uncommon except in children. The nodules may be few or many; are usually small, firm, and non-tender; and are attached to fascia or tendon sheaths over bony prominence such as the elbows, the dorsal surfaces of the hands, the malleoli, the vertebral spines, and the occiput. They persist for days or weeks, are usually recurrent, and are clinically indistinguishable from the nodules or rheumatoid arthritis.

7. **Recurrent nosebleeds:** These may be seen on examination. Recurrent epistaxis are believed by some clinicians to be an indication of 'subclinical' rheumatic fever.

Differential Diagnosis

Rheumatic fever may be confused with the following; rheumatoid arthritis, osteomyelitis, chronic infections, traumatic joint disease, neurocirculatory asthenia or cardiac neurosis, bacterial endocarditis, pulmonary tuberculosis, chronic meningococcemia, meningitis, acute poliomyelitis, connective tissue diseases, serum sickness, drug sensitivity, leukemia, sickle cell anemia, inactive rheumatic heart disease, congenital heart disease, and 'surgical abdomen'.

Complications

Congestive heart failure occurs in severe cases. Other complications include cardiac arrhythmias, pericarditis with large effusion, rheumatic pneumonitis, pulmonary embolism and infarction, cardiac invalidism, and early or late development of permanent heart valve deformity.

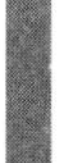

CHRÒNIC CARDIOMYOPATHIES CONGESTIVE IDIOPATHIC OR PRIMARY CARDIOMYOPATHY

This is a miscellaneous group of diseases of unknown cause, divided on the basis of the clinical and hemodynamic features into 3 types; (1) congestive cardiomyopathy, with clinical features of cardiac enlargement, increased cardiac volume, and symptoms and signs of congestive failure with poor pump function; (2) hypertrophic cardiomyopathy and (3) restrictive cardiomyopathy, with infiltrative myocardial disease associated with endomyocardial fibrosis, amyloid disease, scleroderma, hemochromatosis and other disorders that interfere with left ventricular filling and emptying.

Idiopathic congestive cardiomyopathy is a nonspecific diagnosis, and there are no characteristics that differentiate congestive cardiomyopathy from other myocardial disease with a similar end point; congestive failure. Diabetes affects the small vessels of the heart and may be responsible for vasculitis and heart failure and anginal pain similar to those of large vessel coronary disease. The histologically nonspecific nature of fibrosis and hypertrophy of the myocardial fibers has already been noted, and specific causes are unidentified in the great majority of cases.

As newer immunochemical techniques are applied to the investigation of congestive cardiomyopathy, some cases may prove to be of specific immunologic origin. Ten of 40 cases reported from the Cameroons were found to have unsuspected serologic evidence of trypanosomiasis as compared to 2% in a random sample of healthy person in the general population.

Clinical Findings

Symptoms

The disease is suspected early in patients who have dyspnea, chest pain, or palpitations. Dyspnea is typical of that seen in cardiac failure and may progress from dyspnea on exertion to orthopnea, paroxysmal nocturnal dyspnea, and pulmonary edema. When right heart failure supervenes, peripheral edema may be a prominent symptom.

The chest pain is nondescript and not typical of angina pectoris. It may be related to pulmonary congestion or, if pleuritic, to pulmonary embolism. Pericardial pain is rare.

Symptoms of pulmonary or systemic emboli may occur, sometimes dominating the clinical features.

Signs

The signs are those of cardiac hypertrophy or cardiac failure. The cardiac failure is usually left ventricular with pulmonary rales, left ventricular gallop rhythm, and left ventricular heave, which is displaced downward and to the left. If the disease is more advanced, right ventricular enlargement and congestive heart failure are found with a raised venous pressure and pulsating neck veins and liver, an enlarged tender liver, and dependent edema of the legs or sacrum. The signs do not differ from those seen in congestive heart failure from other causes. It is now known whether this is due to the decreased arterial pressure resulting from associated low cardiac output or the development of coronary disease.

Signs of pulmonary emboli or systemic emboli may be found when these complications occur.

Differential Diagnosis

A. **Ischemic Cardiomyopathy:** Increased left ventricular volume with decreased ejection fraction and generalized hypokinesia are seen on left ventricular angiography in both idiopathic cardiomyopathy and ischemic cardiomyopathy. The latter may also be associated with greatly increased cardiac volume, but there are usually segmental defects in contraction rather than symmetrical hpokinesis.

B. **Other Disorders:** Other forms of cardiac disease, hypertension, and secondary cardiomyopathies are discussed elsewhere in this book.

HYPERTROPHIC OBSTRUCTIVE CARDIOMYOPATHY

Classification and Diagnosis

The use of the term hypertrophic obstructive cardiomyopathy to denote the condition described in this section is not entirely satisfactory. It does not suggest any specific cause, although it does identify the two main features of the condition—hypertrophy and obstruction and indicates that the basic cause lies in the heart muscles. The condition may exist with or without obstruction; the former may be provoked by various maneuvers.

Many prefer the terms idiopathic hypertrophic subaortic stenosis or asymmetrical hypertrophy to describe this disease or group of diseases with various causes. The term asymmetrical left ventricular hypertrophy is unsatisfactory both because asymmetry is not in inherent feature of the lesion and because asymmetrical hypertrophy may affect either the septum or the ventricle.

Some patients exhibit features of both congestive and hypertrophic forms. The relationship between hypertrophy and obstruction is also not always clear. Obstruction may be present at all times, may occur intermittently in response to naturally occurring stresses, or may occur only in response to pharmacologic or other stimuli.

The cardinal features of hypertrophic obstructive cardiomyopathy are: The hypertrophy, which involves mainly the septum, interferes with systolic emptying of the left ventricle. The anterior leaflet of the mitral valve comes into apposition with the septal muscle, and narrowing of the outflow tract gives rise to the characteristic systolic murmur. In some cases, septal hypertrophy involves the right side of the heart in addition to or instead of the left, and a picture resembling that of infundibular pulmonary stenosis is then seen.

Cause: The cause of the condition is unknown. In some cases, the disorder is clearly congenital, and familial distribution is also reported. In other cases, the condition appears to develop later in life in a patient with a clear history of essential hypertension.

Age and Sex Incidence: The disease occurs with equal frequency in both sexes and is seen in all age groups. The possibility of associated skeletal muscle disease has been raised.

Criteria for Diagnosis

There is no agreement on what criteria are required for diagnosis. The best evidence of obstruction is a significant pressure difference between the body of the ventricle and the subvalvular area or aorta, using a side-hole closed-tip catheter at left heart catheterization. Systolic anterior motion of the mitral valve on echocardiography is a valuable sign of obstruction, but its specificity is not clear.

Evidence of hypertrophy can also be obtained in different ways. Pathologic examination of the heart is seldom available, and since the obstruction may be 'variable', the state of the heart at autopsy is not necessary relevant. Emptying of the ventricle that is more complete than normal on angiocardiography is an important feature of the disease, but little is known about this aspect of cardiac physiology.

The main problems presented by this clinical entity are in the criteria for diagnosis and in prognosis. Because of the wide variability of the clinical manifestations in different patients, there are wide differences of opinion about the minimum abnormality required to establish the diagnosis. The dangers of creating cardiac neurosis by warning patients with minor or subclinical findings of the possibility of sudden death are obvious.

Clinical Findings

Symptoms

1. **History of heart murmur:** The presence of a heart murmur is not an uncommon reason for referral to a cardiologist. A spurious history of rheumatic fever is sometimes given because the murmur was heard in childhood, perhaps in association with an episode of sore throat.

2. **Dyspnea and chest pain:** Dyspnea on exertion and chest pain are the commonest presenting symptoms. The pain is a dull, aching, substernal discomfort and radiates to the arm like angina pectoris. It resembles the pain in other lesions associated with left ventricular hypertrophy in being closely associated with dyspnea. Classic angina in which there is pain without dyspnea, rapidly relieved by rest and nitroglycerin, is less common. Failure of nitroglycerin to relieve chest pain should suggest the diagnosis of hypertrophic cardiomyopathy.

3. **Other symptoms:** Fatigue, dizziness, and syncope are often reported. The syncope is not necessarily related to the severity of exertion; in fact, it is usually unrelated to exertion and does not carry the dire prognosis that might be expected. Sudden death occurs, especially in familial cases

with marked septal hypertrophy, but the frequency of this outcome is not well documented, and it is not directly related to severity.

4. **Factors influencing symptoms:** The severity of symptoms varies with the state of the circulation. Anything that reduces peripheral resistance, such as a hot environment, pregnancy, standing up suddenly, exercise, or amyl nitrite inhalation may induce or exaggerate outflow obstruction and bring on symptoms. Left ventricular failure occurs late and may follow the onset of atrial fibrillation. Congestive heart failure occurs but is quite uncommon.

Signs

1. **Pulse:** The pulse is jerky, with a bifid quality. The rapid initial upstroke is followed by a small tidal wave. The outflow obstruction develops after the start of systole, and the initial ejection of blood through an unobstructed outflow tract is responsible for the sharp rise in the pulse wave. The characteristic pulse should arouse the physician's suspicion when it occurs in conjunction with cardiac failure or a relatively low arterial pressure.

2. **Cardiac impulse:** The same mechanism accounts for the findings on palpation at the apex of the heart in some cases, where a bifid impulse is felt during systole. In other cases, the apical impulse is bifid for another reason. This produces a palpable presystolic impulse that gives a double apical impulse. When both of these factors are present, there is a *triple cardiac impulse* that is virtually pathognomonic of the condition.

3. **Systolic murmur:** There is almost invariably a harsh, long systolic murmur that peaks like other ejection, murmurs in mid systole but starts early and may last for almost the whole of systole.

4. **Other signs:** Third and fourth heart sounds are commonly heard, but ejection clicks and aortic diastolic murmurs are quite rare. Mitral incompetence is also present in many

cases, making it difficult to decide whether the murmur is pansystolic or ejection in character. Posture has a marked effect on the murmur, and sudden squatting often abolishes or lessens the intensity of the murmur, as it does the obstruction. The Valsalva maneuver increases the murmurs of mitral regurgitation and of obstruction to the outflow of the left ventricle by decreasing the size of the left ventricle as a result of the reduced venous return.

5. **Effect of an ectopic beat:** The peripheral arterial blood pressure is often smaller after a long diastolic pause following an ectopic beat. The more forceful ventricular contraction increases the degree of outflow obstruction.

6. **Effect of amyl nitrite:** Amyl nitrite inhalation and isoproterenol induce or exaggerate the outflow obstruction murmur, whereas phenylephrine relieves obstruction. Such studies may help in determining the degree of associated mitral incompetence. Amyl nitrite also brings out the murmur of aortic stenosis, but murmur is shorter and associated with a slowly rising pulse and should not lead to confusion.

Differential Diagnosis

The physical signs of hypertrophic obstructive cardiomyopathy resemble those of mitral incompetence or ventricular septal defect more closely than those of aortic stenosis. There is, however, left ventricular outflow obstruction in both valvular and subvalvular lesions, and although the jerky, bifid pulse of obstructive cardiomyopathy is readily distinguished from the anacrotic, slow rising pulse of aortic stenosis, this lesion does enter into the differential diagnosis in practice. Marked left ventricular hypertrophy is not seen in mitral incompetence or ventricular septal defect, and its presence in a patient with

a long, harsh systolic murmur should suggest obstructive cardiomyopathy.

Complications

Atrial fibrillation, ventricular arrhythmias, and sudden death are important complications, and a relationship is presumed to exist between the latter two. Young patients with the familial disease seem most prone to these complications. It may possibly be related to ventricular arrhythmias or conduction defects. No reliable predictors of sudden death have been discovered, although one-third of patients who died suddenly had been taking propranolol, but the adequacy of the dose can be questioned. Left ventricular failure with pulmonary edema may follow the onset of atrial fibrillation. In other cases, left ventricular failure may actually relieve obstruction and help to improve the condition because it leads to cardiac dilatation. Mitral incompetence may be caused by long-term damage to the valve by turbulent flow in the outflow tract. Endocardial fibrosis and thickening are seen in this area and are thought to be due to mechanical trauma.

■ RESTRICTIVE CARDIOMYOPATHY

Restrictive cardiomyopathy constitutes the third general category of Goodwin's classification of cardiomyopathy and is the least common variety. This variant frequently shades into the category of hypertrophic cardiomyopathy because the hypertrophic changes of the latter may decrease compliance of the ventricles and simulate some of the findings of restrictive cardiomyopathy. The term "restrictive" is used because a characteristic feature of the condition is a restriction in ventricular filling resulting from a non-compliant, less distensible ventricle. An infiltrative pathologic process is responsible for the decreased compliance and other clinical features.

Chapter 7

Pericarditis

Pericardium though not essential for life has roles to play in both health and disease.

DIFFERENTIAL DIAGNOSIS

Enlargement of the heart due to dilatation or hypertrophy is virtually the only condition, which must be distinguished from pericardial effusion, although primary tumor (angiosarcoma) may rarely enter into the differential diagnosis. In some cases, there may be effusion in addition to cardiac enlargement. In these cases, the introduction of air into the pericardium at the time of pericardiocentesis serves to indicate heart size and the thickness of the pericardium. Echocardiographic examination has provided significant help in differentiating between pericardial effusion and cardiac enlargement.

COMPLICATIONS

Cardiac tamponade is the most important complication of pericardial effusion. It can occur with surprising speed, because the compliance of the pericardial cavity can be markedly nonlinear, and the accumulation of a small additional amount of fluid can cause a marked rise in intrapericardial pressure. Close monitoring of the systemic venous pressure, either clinically or via a catheter and manometer in severely ill patients, is the best means of detecting the development of this complication. Fibrosis and thickening of the pericardium almost inevitably accompany or follow effusion, and the possibility of seroconstriction must always be borne in mind.

CARDIAC TAMPONADE

The time necessary for fluid to accumulate in the pericardial cavity can vary from seconds (in rupture of a major structure) to weeks or months in chronic infections. The rate of rise of intrapericardial pressure is the most important factor in determining the development of the hemodynamic and clinical features of cardiac tamponade. When the fluid accumulates rapidly, or if effusion occurs into a pericardium thickened and noncompliant because of fibrosis, serious interference with cardiac filling can occur with remarkable speed. The compliance of the pericardial cavity is markedly nonlinear, so that although significant amounts of fluid can sometimes accumulate without much rise in pressure, a further slight increase in fluid may produce a considerable rise in pressure as well as symptoms and signs of cardiac tamponade.

Cardiac tamponade develops when the pressure in the pericardial cavity rises to a level equal to that in the heart during diastole. Because the right atrium and ventricle have the lowest diastolic pressure, they are the first structures to be compressed by the increasing pericardial pressure. The venous pressure and the intracardiac and intrapericardial pressures then rise together as pericardial tamponade progresses, and soon the diastolic pressures in both the left and right sides of the heart are raised. At this stage, respiration has a marked hemodynamic effect, and pulsus paradoxus develops. The increased negative intrathoracic pressure produced by inspiration stretches the right heart and opens up the compressed right ventricle, increasing its output and filling the lungs with blood. In severe cases, the interventricular septum may bulge to the left on inspiration. All these events interfere with left ventricular filling and cause an inspiratory fall in arterial pressure and left ventricular output. Conversely, on expiration, the right ventricular volume decreases and the blood stored in the lungs returns to the left heart, increasing its output. The reciprocal effects of inspiration and expiration on the right and left heart are not seen when there is an atrial septal defect, nor do they occur unless the diastolic pressures in both sides of the heart are equal. Thus, pulsus paradoxus is not seen when the left ventricle is hypertrophied and stiff, as occurs in some cases of chronic renal disease and hypertension; in these instances, left atrial pressure is higher than right atrial pressure, and the right ventricle is compressed before the left heart is.

Clinical Findings

Symptoms

Acute cardiac tamponade may cause symptoms ranging from anxiety, sweating, dyspnea, dizziness and syncope to frank shock. The clinical picture ranges from slight circulatory and hemodynamic abnormalities to circulatory collapse. The precise point at which tamponade can be said to have occurred is difficult to clinically.

Signs

Venous pressure is raised in cardiac tamponade because the right heart cannot accommodate all the inspiratory increase in venous return, and the venous pressure rises (Kussmaul's sign). The rise in pericardial pressure interferes with cardiac filling throughout the whole of the cardiac cycle, and the rapid Y descent seen in the jugular venous pulse in pericardial constriction is absent. The cardiac impulse is classically not palpable, the heart sounds are distant, and murmurs are absent. Since filling is impaired throughout diastole, the rapid filling phase of early diastole seen in pericardial constriction is not prominent, and a pericardial third sound ("knock") is seldom heard.

The pulse rate is rapid, and the blood pressure and pulse pressure are low. Pulsus paradoxus defined as a fall of more than 10 mm Hg or 10% in systolic arterial blood pressure on normal inspiration, can be detected when the blood pressure is measured either indirectly or directly. The term pulsus paradoxus is a misnomer because the condition is basically an exaggeration of the normal finding of a decrease in arterial pressure with inspiration and therefore is not actually "paradoxical".

Differential Diagnosis

Cardiac tamponade must be distinguished from other acute cardiac emergencies such as hemorrhage, myocardial infarction, and pulmonary embolism. Signs of a falling arterial pressure and cardiac output and a rising venous pressure and heart rate should alert the physician to the possibility of cardiac tamponade, and pulsus paradoxus strongly suggests the diagnosis. Echocardiography is the most helpful diagnostic investigation.

Complications

The complications of cardiac tamponade include those of circulatory collapse, with inadequate perfusion of any organ system, but most commonly the brain and the kidneys. Early recognition and prompt treatment are essential, especially in acute cases.

PERICARDIAL CONSTRICTION

The term pericardial constriction is used to describe both the classic chronic disease (constrictive pericarditis that mimics right heart failure, and the subacute condition, in which a rigid pericardium and pericardial fluid combine to compress the heart and interfere with its late diastolic filing (subacute effusive constrictive pericarditis). With the improved diagnostic techniques now available, more subacute cases are being recognized, especially tuberculosis, the principal cause of chronic pericardial constriction. Viral, uremic, neoplastic and traumatic (including irradiation) pericardial diseases are more likely to cause the subacute form than classic chronic constrictive pericarditis, in which no evidence of effusion is ordinarily detectable.

The chronic inflammatory changes in the pericardial cavity surround the heart with a sheath of tough, unyielding fibrous tissue that interferes with cardiac filling. The actual, or effective, intrapericardial pressure rises and the pressure in all heart chambers at the end of diastole rises. The heart is immobilized because it is encased in an unyielding fibrous cage that interferes with its excursion during contraction and relaxation. The more compliant chambers, the atria and the right ventricle, bear the brunt of the burden, but end-diastolic pressures in all cardiac chambers tend to be the same: about 1.5–25 mm Hg in severe cases.

The encasement does not necessarily involve all chambers but the effective intrapericardial pressure rises on both sides of the heart. Although the effects of the disease are more severe in the more distensible right heart, the left side is almost invariably involved also.

Clinical Findings

Symptoms

Swelling of the abdomen and legs is the symptoms suggesting a diagnosis of constrictive pericarditis. Dyspnea is not generally prominent but it is usually present in all cases to some degree. Anorexia, weakness, wasting and dyspepsia are seen in advanced cases. These symptoms are due to a combination of low cardiac output and marked hepatic congestion. A history of a precious attack of acute or subacute pericarditis is an important feature. The absence of a history of the other forms of heart disease is also valuable. Pain is not a prominent feature of the disease. The patient is usually able to lie flat without any problem and does not suffer from paroxysmal nocturnal dyspnea.

Signs

The pulse is usually rapid and the blood pressure low. Pulsus paradoxus is less common in constrictive pericarditis as compared to tamponade unless constrictive pericarditis is associated with effusion. The heartbeat is irregular in about 30% of cases because of atrial fibrillation. The onset of arrhythmia is related to the age of the patient and the severity of the disease.

The patient appears chronically ill in advanced cases. the neck veins are distended, the venous pressure is markedly raised and there is a rapid Y descent. Tamponade and constriction cannot be differentiated on the basis of a consistent difference in venous pulse. Venous pressure and the nature of the venous pulse are important in pericardial constriction. The neck veins usually show a major negative wave at the time of the Y descent . This constitutes diastolic collapse of the veins and is caused by rapid filling of the right heart in early diastole at a time when intracardiac pressure is at its lowest after the end of systole. The sign is not specific for pericardial disease and can be seen in any form of severe right heart failure. Another nonspecific physical sign associated with pericardial disease is Kussmaul's sign, an inspiratory increase in venous pressure. When right heart filling is excessive, the increase in venous pressure occurring on inspiration cannot be accommodated in the restricted pericardial constriction, cardiac filling stops abruptly when the heart meets the limits of the unyielding pericardial cavity. This shock is felt as a palpable diastolic impulse in some cases. It is associated with the pericardial "knock", or filling sound, that generally occurs before the usual third sound. It can be the loudest sound in the cardiac cycle. There is usually no murmur and the heart sounds are soft.

Rales may be present at the base of the lung and the liver is usually markedly enlarged and tender but non-pulsating. Ascites tends to be more prominent than ankle edema (ascites precox) and the combination of wasting edema resemblances that seen in the cirrhosis of liver.

Differential Diagnosis

Superior vena caval obstruction should not be confused with constrictive pericarditis because venous pulsation and evidence of inferior vena caval obstruction, with hepatic enlargement and ascites, are absent. Similarly, cirrhosis of the liver, in which the jugular venous pressure is not raised, should be readily distinguished. The principal entities with which constrictive pericarditis can be confused are restrictive cardiomyopathy and endomyocardial fibrosis. The distinction is extremely difficult to make; furthermore, pericardial, myocardial and endocardial fibrosis tend to influence one another because the fibrotic process tends to spread from one structure to the other. Pericardial fibrosis tends to involve the muscle of the thin-walled right ventricle; similarly, endocardial fibrosis tends to spread to the underlying cardiac muscle. Although exploration may be indicated in difficult cases, it is harmful in patients with cardiomyopathy and should be avoided if possible.

The response to treatment with digitals and its derivatives can be helpful. The venous pressure may fall to normal in patients with right heart failure. In contrast, in constrictive pericarditis, the venous pressure remains high in spite of medical therapy.

Complications

Involvement of the myocardium is such an inevitable consequence of pericardial constriction that it can hardly be called a complication. The effects are most clearly seen after surgery, when the heart (especially the right ventricle) may dilate when the constricting pericardium is removed, with subsequent cardiac dilation and failure.

Chapter 8

Pulmonary Heart Diseases

■ INTRODUCTION

Cor pulmonale is the condition of affection of right ventricle secondary to lung disease with or without right ventricular failure.

The principal site of involvement in pulmonary heart disease is the pulmonary vascular bed. The pulmonary blood vessels, arterioles, capillaries and veins may be affected by heart disease, leading to cardiac involvement, mainly affecting the right heart. The pulmonary blood vessels themselves may be the primary site of disease, as in schistosomiasis (bilharziasis), primary pulmonary hypertension, pulmonary arteriovenous fistula, or the lodging of emboli in the pulmonary vessels, which interrupts blood supply to the lungs and affects the function of either the right or the left heart. The presence of heart disease has an important effect on the response of the lungs to embolization. The lungs have a double arterial blood supply from bronchial and pulmonary arteries. In normal persons, the lungs do not become infarcted when their pulmonary arterial blood supply is occluded. When the lungs are congested, as is commonly the case in patients with heart disease, pulmonary embolism is followed by pulmonary infarction, leading to hemorrhagic consolidation with obvious pulmonary parenchymal involvement.

The close relationship between heart disease and lung disease is further emphasizes by the effects of cigarette smoking. Carcinoma of the bronchus and pulmonary emphysema are closely associated with excessive cigarette smoking. Premature coronary artery disease is also more common in habitual cigarette smokers. Thus, both the heart and lung diseases are often present in the same patient and since dyspnea and chest pain are important symptoms in both heart and lung diseases, diagnostic problems, especially cause of total disability between disease of the heart and disease of the lungs, are particularly frequent.

Pulmonary Hypertension

The development of increased pulmonary arterial pressure (pulmonary hypertension) represents the most important response of pulmonary blood vessels to disease. Pulmonary hypertension may be result from primary parenchymal disease of the lungs, from changes in the walls of the blood vessels, or from obstruction to the lumen by thrombosis or embolization to the lumen caused by thrombosis or embolization. The clinical picture varies widely depending on the cause of the pulmonary vascular involvement, but the final common pathway tends to result in right ventricular overload, right ventricular hypertrophy, and right heart failure. The term "cor pulmonale" is used to describe right heart involvement, and cor pulmonale is said to be present when any right sided abnormality can be demonstrated; Frank right heart failure does not have to be present.

Pulmonary circulation in the adult seems to be almost completely passive when compared to the systemic circulation. It behaves as an unreactive, low pressure, low resistance, short, high flow pathway from the heart via the pulmonary arteries to the pulmonary capillary bed, which constitutes the large (100 m²) site of gas exchange. The fetal, neonatal and infant pulmonary circulations are less passive and have higher pressure and resistances in relation to their corresponding systemic circulations.

Primary Pulmonary Hypertension

In rare cases, pulmonary arterial vasoconstriction occurs without a rise in left atrial pressure, giving rise to a disease known as primary, or idiopathic, pulmonary hypertension. The condition is commonest in premenopausal women but can occur at any age. The onset is insidious and the course usually relentlessly progressive, leading to death in 2–8 years from intractable right heart failure. The most striking clinical feature is low cardiac output, with weakness, fatigue, dyspnea, palpitations and edema and ascites development as right heart failure progresses. Cyanosis is often present and may be peripheral, owing to low output or rarely, central, in cases in which diffuse fine pulmonary fibrosis (which does not show up on the chest X-ray) interferes with gas exchange. Syncope on effort can occasionally occur. At autopsy, the abnormal pulmonary vascular bed is so frequently seen to be the site of thrombosis and embolism that some have doubted the primary vasospastic nature of this condition.

Thromboembolic pulmonary hypertension can occur as a separate identifiable disease in patients who have repeated episodes of pulmonary embolism that are so frequent that complete resolution does not have time to occur between attacks. It is difficult to differentiate between vasospasm and thromboembolism in the genesis of primary pulmonary hypertension because multiple small pulmonary emboli can trigger reflex changes and may also produce pulmonary vasoconstriction. Pulmonary embolism is seldom the sole cause of chronic pulmonary hypertension but undoubtedly often contributes significantly to the clinical in patients with mixed lesions.

Right Heart Failure Secondary to Lung Disease

The ultimate result of pulmonary vascular disease is right heart failure. This may be acute, as in massive pulmonary embolism; subacute, as when an acute pulmonary infection occurs in a patient with pre-existing moderate pulmonary hypertension; or chronic, as in the end stages of chronic lung disease or primary pulmonary hypertension. The clinical picture varies with the cause of the lung disease and pulmonary thromboembolism constitutes an important variable factor. The name cor pulmonale has been used to describe the condition, but this term should be used to cover any form of right-sided ventricular abnormality due to lung disease.

Massive Pulmonary Embolism: Acute Right Heart Failure (Acute Cor Pulmonale)

Acute cor pulmonale is seen almost exclusively in association with massive pulmonary embolism. Massive pulmonary embolism usually occurs in apparently healthy persons who may be of any age. The disease affects females more often than males. Patients have usually been recently subject to some minor trauma recent normal delivery, hernia operation, minor gynecologic or urologic surgery, varicose vein operation, or some other procedure involving the legs or pelvis is ordinarily the precipitating factor. Loosely adherent, soft, friable thrombus forms undetected in the veins of the legs or pelvis (phlebothrombosis). The thrombus suddenly breaks loose (in classic cases during straining at stool) and lodges at or near the bifurcation of the main pulmonary artery. The patient complains of sudden, severe central chest pain and collapses, often with loss of consciousness. Death can occur within a few minutes, if the thrombus is large and does not dislodge. If the thrombus is smaller or moves more peripherally, either spontaneously or in response to pounding on the chest or closed chest massage, acute cor pulmonale rather than sudden death is seen, and the condition may run a subacute course.

Dyspnea, cyanosis, anxiety, impaired consciousness and all the manifestations of an acute circulatory catastrophe are present. The diagnosis is difficult to confirm in the face of simultaneous emergency and supportive treatment and the general hectic activity involved in managing an acute life-threatening situation. Physical examination may not reveal any specific diagnostic signs.

Clinical Findings

Symptoms

The classic symptoms of a chest pain that is often worse on inspiration, dyspnea, cough and hemoptysis in susceptible patients such as those with congestive heart failure, mitral valve disease, or myocardial infarction should strongly suggest a diagnosis of pulmonary embolism. Not infrequently, unexplained dyspnea, fever, tachycardia, increase in venous pressure, or worsening of venous congestion provides acute to the diagnosis, but in many cases the acute episode passes unnoticed.

Signs

Physical signs in the lungs depend on the development of consolidation or pleural involvement. Pleural friction rub, impaired movement, dullness to percussion, diminished air entry and bronchial breathing can be heard and signs of pleural effusion may develop such increased right ventricular impulse, increased intensity of the pulmonary valve closure sound, or palpable pulmonary artery pulsation should be sought.

Differential Diagnosis

The diagnosis of pulmonary embolism can be extremely difficult, especially in patients who are ill from other causes and in postoperative patients. The condition is so insidious that it should be suspected in any sick patient in whom unexplained deterioration of failure to thrive is detected. The physician must maintain a high index of suspicion in order to make the correct diagnosis. In many cases, the diagnosis can be made in retrospect from careful examination of the chart of the vital signs. A sudden increase in heart rate of respiratory rate, followed by an unexplained rise in temperature on the following day, may have occurred in a patient with an obvious pulmonary infarct that was not previously apparent. Intercurrent lower respiratory tract infections can be readily mistaken for pulmonary emboli and vice versa. Likewise, minor, short-lived episodes of acute pulmonary congestion may cause a similar clinical picture. Repeated episodes of embolism tend to differ slightly in their manifestations, whereas recurrent pulmonary congestion tends to produce a series of similar episodes.

Pulmonary embolism enters into the differential diagnosis of almost all forms of lung disease and many varieties of heart disease. It occurs during the course of these diseases and may also be confused with diseases themselves. Thus, pneumonia, atelectasis (especially if they occur postoperatively), and pleurisy with or without effusion may all be confused with pulmonary infarction. Hemorrhage into the lung is an important feature of pulmonary infarction that is also seen in other conditions such as bronchial carcinoma, tuberculosis, or any disease causing hemoptysis. Acute chest pain in pulmonary embolism can be confused with that occurring myocardial infarction, spontaneous pneumothorax, pericarditis, aortic dissection, and even upper abdominal disease such as cholecystitis or perforated perptic ulcer.

▌ RIGHT HEART FAILURE SECONDARY TO CHRONIC LUNG DISEASE

Pulmonary hypertension ultimately leads to right heart failure. the clinical picture depends primarily on the cause of the lung disease.

Chronic cor pulmonale is defined as heart disease (rather than heart failure) that is secondary to disease of the lung/part of respiratory system. Right ventricular enlargement secondary to chronic disease of the respiratory system is most commonly due to parenchymal lung disease such as fibrosis, emphysema or pneumonia. The clinical picture is little influenced by the underlying cause, which may be pulmonary granuloma, sarcoidosis, scleroderma, pneumoconiosis, or any form of fibrosis, including idiopathic lesions (Hamman-Rich disease). The clinical picture is usually one of recurrent episodes of pulmonary infection of bronchial obstruction leading to temporary increases in the load on the right heart and right heart failure. Any lesion producing alveolar hypoxia causes a vicious cycle because of increased pulmonary arterial pressure due to pulmonary vasoconstriction. This mechanism is involved in alveolar hypoventilation due to weakness or paralysis of the respiratory muscles and also in central nervous disease leading to inadequate pulmonary ventilation. Both these conditions can cause chronic cor pulmonale even when the lungs themselves are normal. Massive obesity, as in the Pickwickian syndrome, can also cause right heart failure; it is another cause of alveolar hypoventilation in which the lungs are normal. Chest wall disorders such as kyphosis and scoliosis may occasionally lead to heart failure but usually only when chest infection is present. Before antibiotic therapy and assisted ventilation were available, the first episode of right heart failure was often fatal in patients who had chronic lung disease secondary to respiratory infection or obstruction. Modern treatment of acute pulmonary failure often leads to recovery but leaves the lungs damaged to a variable degree and often more vulnerable to a recurrent episode of infection. After several episodes of acute right heart failure, the patient reaches a precarious condition in which even minor illnesses such as influenza of an upper respiratory infection can be life-threatening. In such patients, the degree of right heart failure is an indication of the stage of the disease. Arterial hypoxia increases cardiac output by causing systemic vasodilatation and especially by increasing the heart rate. These factors tend to aggravate right heart failure. Since patients with chronic lung disease is common and an element of left heart failure is frequently present in addition to right heart failure. Some feel that right heart failure can lead to left heart failure as the enlarging right ventricle displaces the left ventricle backwards, but this is difficult to prove.

Clinical Findings

Symptoms

Dyspnea is the primary symptom in patients with chronic cor pulmonale. Coexisting pulmonary and cardiac disease may take it difficult to determine the cause of dyspnea is most commonly due to the increased work of breathing resulting from the mechanical effects of the lung disease causing the right heart overload.

However, dyspnea is also seen in the rarest form of chronic cor pulmonale—primary pulmonary hypertension. In this condition, the mechanical properties of the lungs are normal and some other explanation must be sought to explain the dyspnea. An inadequate systemic cardiac output is thought to cause alveolar hyperventilation and excessive ventilation, especially during exercise, is thought to be responsible for the dyspnea. Edema of the ankles, abdominal swelling and right upper quadrant pain due to hepatic congestion are often seen. Palpitations, weakness, syncope and coldness of the hands and feet also occur in primary pulmonary hypertension.

Signs

Noncardiac signs: Patients with arterial hypoxia due to bronchits tend to exhibit hypervolemia and vasodilation rather the vasoconstriction and low output state seen in patients with emphysema and primary pulmonary hypertension. Patients with chronic lung disease have been divided into "blue bloaters" where, hypoxia, hypervolemia, recurrent bronchitis, and cor pulmonale are prominent, and "pink puffers", in whom hypoxia is absent, hypovolemia and emphysema are common and cor pulmonale is rare. Similarly, cor pulmonale has been classified as either hypoxic or pulmonary hypertensive, depending on whether a high output or a low output state predominates. Such generalizations involved but must not be taken as definitely, mutually exclusive categories.

Cyanosis and clubbing of the fingers are often seen. Then cyanosis may be peripheral, due to the low cardiac output in patients with pulmonary hypertension or central and associated with significant arterial hypoxemia ($PO_0 < 60$ mm Hg) and hypercapnia ($PCO_2 > 50$ mm Hg) in patients with chronic lung disease or alveolar hypoventilation. Clubbing of the fingers is most frequently seen in patients with chronic pulmonary infections or bronchial carcinoma. Tachycardia and a raised jugular venous pressure with a and v waves occur. Hepatomegaly, ascites and edema of the ankles are seen if the patient is in right heart failure.

Cardiac signs: Cardiac manifestation depends on the nature of the lung disease. In patients with emphysema, bronchitis or bronchial obstruction, the cardiac impulse may be difficult to palpate because of overlying lung tissue. The sounds may be distant and murmurs absent. Conversely, in primary pulmonary hypertension, a prominent right ventricular heave below the sternum, a loud pulmonary valve closure component of a closely split second heart sound and ejection click and a short pulmonary diastolic (Graham Steell) murmur due to pulmonary incompetence. In later stages, a pansystolic high-pitched murmur of tricuspid incompetence is often easily detected.

Differential Diagnosis

Disorders to be differential from right heart failure due to lung disease include mitral stenosis, thromboembolic pulmonary hypertension and Eisenmeneger's syndrome. When coincidental pulmonary disease is present, the differential diagnosis can be extremely difficult. Cardiac catheterization is indicated when clear evidence of pulmonary hypertension is found. This diagnosis is suspected more commonly than it is proved and clinical signs of right heart failure (palpable pulmonary arterial pulsation and loud pulmonary valve closure) tend to be unreliable signs of pulmonary hypertension.

Complications

Right heart failure is such an integral part of chronic cor pulmonale that it is hardly a complication. Similarly, chest infection, pulmonary thrombosis, embolism and alveolar hypoxia occur so frequently in the course of the disease that they are not really considered complications. Atrial arrhythmias are relatively common in acute exacerbations of pulmonary infection, but chronic atrial fibrillation is rare. Pulmonary valvular incompetence causing an immediate diastolic (Graham Steell) murmur over the pulmonary artery is more a part of the disease than a complication.

DIFFERENTIATION OF HEART DISEASE AND LUNG DISEASE

Lung disease and heart disease often coexist. The harmful effects of cigarette smoking predispose to chronic bronchitis and emphysema and also to carcinoma of the bronchus. They also increase the risk of premature coronary artery disease. In consequence, many patients suffer from both cardiac and pulmonary diseases, and the two compound one another. The hypoxia associated with acute exacerbations of chronic obstructive lung disease increases the cardiac output and increases the cardiac output and increases the load on the heart, which may be already compromised by coronary disease. Conversely, myocardial infarction or left heart failure in a patient with impaired pulmonary function due to emphysema predisposes to acute pulmonary infection leading to pulmonary failure (hypoxia and hypercapnia). Whereas the distinction between pure lung disease and heart disease is relatively easy, separating the pulmonary and cardiac elements in mixed lesions is extremely difficult.

Clinical Findings

Symptoms

Breathlessness is an important symptom in both heart and lung diseases. The dyspnea of lung disease tends to be episodic, being worse at some times than others. It is not infrequently present at rest, when attacks of asthma, bronchospasm or acute bronchitis occur. It may also be worse on exercise, especially when asthma or bronchospasm is induced by effort. The dyspnea of emphysema produces a basic, permanent, irreversible level of dyspnea. Although the patient's dyspnea may be worse at times, it never remits completely. It is thus important in obtaining a history of dyspnea on the patient's breathlessness varies from day to day and to concentrate on the level of dyspnea on the patient's "best day". If significant emphysema is present, dyspnea will be present even on the "best day". Conversely, if the patient has a normal exercise tolerance on the best day, then emphysema is not present. The dyspnea of lung disease is associated with the application of increased force to move the lungs and thorax and the patient is aware of the mechanical problem in breathing.

Chest pain occurs in both heart and lung disease. The patient with lung disease complains of a tight constricting feeling across the chest on exertion or at rest usually be distinguished from angina pain, because it is discomfort rather than pain and usually neither radiation like angina nor is so quantitatively related to exertion. Pleural pain when suggests lung disease but can occur in heart disease when pulmonary embolism leads to pulmonary infarction.

Cough occurs in both heart and lung. Its disease presence is much more common in lung diseases, but pulmonary congestion secondary to raised left atrial pressure can also cause cough. The cough in heart disease is dry and unproductive unless pulmonary edema develops, when profuse watery or frothy sputum occurs. The cough of pulmonary congestion often comes on with exercise. Cough with purulent, mucopurulent, rusty or tenacious sputum is indicative of lung diseases. Hemoptysis occurs in both the heart and lung disease and its presence is not often of value in distinguishing heart and lung diseases.

Signs

In comparison with symptoms, there is much less overlap in physical signs of heart and lung diseases. Pleural friction rubs and rales and rhonchi can occur in both. The pulmonary congestion and edema can be mistaken for those of asthma or bronchospasm, but "cardiac asthma" is not often confused with asthma or bronchitis because of the history of previous attacks in asthma and the presence of obvious signs of mitral or left ventricular disease in patients with pulmonary congestion.

Arterial blood gas measurement should be made if there is any doubt. The hypoxia (PO_2 < 70 mm Hg, PCO_2 > 45 mm Hg) often seen in lung disease are rare in heart disease except when pulmonary edema is present. In difficult cases, cardiac catheterization with measurement of pulmonary vascular resistance and full pulmonary function studies are likely to be needed to separate the effects of lung disease from those of heart disease.

Chapter 9

Some other Clinically Important Cardiovascular Conditions

CARDIAC TUMORS

Cardiac tumors are more frequently metastatic than primary. The state of the primary tumor is most often in lung or the breast, indicating that the tumor is likely to spread locally to involve the heart or pericardium. Various types of lymphoma also tend to involve the heart, again mainly by spread from the mediastinum. Metastases seldom affect left ventricular function, although when pericardial effusion occurs, the patient may show manifestations of pericardial tamponade. The most common primary malignant tumors involving the heart are sarcomas. The most common benign tumor is a myxoma usually left atrial myxoma—although the right may be involved and more rarely, the ventricle.

A cardiac tumor obstructs blood flow in the region of the heart may interfere with atrial or ventricular filling, either within or outside the cardiac chambers; or may involve the pericardium.

Clinical Findings

Symptoms: The presenting symptoms in patients with cardiac tumors are often bizarre and confusing. Posturally variable dyspnea, cough and syncope of systemic or pulmonary congestion with dyspnea or edema are sometimes seen. In patients with metastases, there is often no clinical clue to involvement of the heart in the patients' history.

Signs: Evidence of pericardial involvement may be found with pericardial friction or increased venous pressure. In myxoma, there are often changing murmurs, perhaps influenced by posture. The tumor is often pedunculated and is mobile and the degree of obstruction to blood flow varies with posture and varying hemodynamic events. The patients may thus have a diastolic murmur in one body position but not in another. Careful search for evidence of embolism is always important and the recovery of embolic material for histologic examination is sometimes of diagnostic value. In some cases of myxoma, systemic signs such as fever, tachycardia and clubbing of the fingers are seen. Echocardiography is very useful.

Differential Diagnosis

Left atrial myxoma is most likely to be confused with rheumatic disease of the mitral valve. The episodic nature of the symptoms and signs and the presence of systemic manifestation are the most useful features in diagnosis. Other primary or secondary tumors involving the heart can be confused with pericardial disease with myocarditis or cardiomyopathy or with valvular heart disease in some instances. The systemic manifestation of myxoma brings to mind many differential diagnoses, e.g. infective endocarditis, connective tissue disorders, occult malignancy and chronic infections.

Hypotension

Hypotension should be regarded as a symptom rather than a disease. Since gravity is the most significant force affecting the cardiovascular system, it is not surprising that hypotension is ordinarily more apparent when the patient stands upright and that the compensatory mechanism maintaining arterial pressure are more severely stressed in the standing than in the recumbent position.

Causes of Hypotension

Hypotension results from inadequate cardiac output, as in myocardial infarction; from inadequate circulating blood volume; or from failure of the normal reflex mechanism that maintain a constant arterial pressure. All these factors operate in number of disorders and several may combine in a given patient to cause the primary symptom of hypotension—dizziness or faintness—which is made worse when the patient suddenly stands up.

Disturbances of blood volume are clinically more common than disturbances of reflex control of the circulation and they stem from two factors. One is a decrease in plasma or red cell volume due to hemorrhage, dehydration, excessive diuresis or excessive sweating; the other is a change in capacity of a blood-filled compartment (heart, arteries, capillaries or veins).

Decreased blood volume as a cause of hypotension is particularly striking in adrenal insufficiency disorders, e.g. Addison's disease and hypopituitarism. Wasting disorders of the bowel associated with diarrhea and anemia are also commonly associated with hypotension and a sudden episode of faintness with hypotension is often the first manifestation of gastrointestinal hemorrhage.

Abnormalities of reflex control of arterial pressure usually result from disease of the central nervous system and its autonomic pathways. Disease may also affect the peripheral parts of the autonomic nervous system via innervations of blood vessels that are particularly susceptible to the effect of drugs.

Clinical Features

The clinical picture of hypotension associated with an inadequate blood volume is dominated by the effects of the compensatory mechanisms that are medicated by the autonomic nervous system. These effects cause anxiety, weakness, palpitations, tachycardia, restlessness, vasoconstriction, sweating, pallor and cold extremities. In contrast, in hypotension associated with autonomic nervous system disease, the patient faints with few or no accompanying symptoms. Dizziness and dimness of vision usually give little warning of impending loss of consciousness. Recovery is rapid when cerebral blood flow is restored with the patient in the recumbent position.

Hypotension Associated with Inadequate Blood Volume

A. **Vasovagal Attacks and Fainting:** The commonest form of hypotension is that seen in simple fainting. A sudden muscular vasodilatation medicated by cholinergic sympathetic nerves results in an acute fall in effective blood volume owing to sudden pooling of blood in peripheral areas of the body (normally the legs). Simple fainting occurs in normal subjects and may also be provoked by disease, especially myocardial infarction with or without pain. Fainting may also occur during cardiologic investigation. The vagus nerve plays an important part in the mechanism of fainting and simple faints are sometimes called vagal attacks. The primary stimulus to simple fainting may be physical or psychic. Trauma, pain or stimulation of vagal afferents especially in the ascending aorta near the right coronary ostium may cause hypotension, even in recumbent subjects. Fear, the sight of blood, observing trauma to others or seeing other people faint may all cause hypotension. Premonitory symptoms include feeling alternately hot and cold, yawning, sweating and an uneasy or sinking feeling in the epigastrium. The patient looks pale and develops bradycardia before the ultimate sudden acute muscular vasodilatation.

Neurocirculatory Asthenia (Cardiac Neurosis)

The functional cardiac disorder known as neurocirculatory asthenia is also called effort syndrome, disordered action of the heart, Soldier's heart and Da Costa's syndrome. This condition causes the most difficulty during wartime, apparently healthy men who develop symptoms either during military training or during actual combat that make them entirely unfit for the military service. A similar clinical picture is seen in civilian life, but in that context the symptoms vary from patient to patient and the four classic symptoms of dyspnea, palpitations, chest pain and fatigue seen in wartime are supplemented by other complaints.

Clinical Findings

The spectrum of cases is wide, with incapacity varying from mild to severe. The condition has usually been present before military service and is found in men, women and children. Wood stressed the psychological aspects of the disorder and considered the condition to be a form of anxiety neurosis. Physician sometimes unwittingly contribute to the patients with heart disease. The patient becomes fearful of exercise and the combination of anxiety and inactivity is particularly likely to produce the clinical picture of cardiac neurosis. Occasionally, prolonged enforced bed rest in suspected cases of rheumatic fever may lead to cardiac neurosis. The physician must guard against the possibility of causing or aggravating neurotic tendencies, especially in young persons.

Symptoms: Dyspnea on exertion or on exposure to threatening situations is the most predominant symptom and all symptoms are aggravated by mental or physical stress. The breathlessness often involves an inability to get a deep enough or satisfying breath. Other symptoms, in the order of frequency are weakness, palpitations,

noncardiac pain in the left chest, fatigue, cold sweating (especially of the palms), nervousness, dizziness, headache, tremulousness, sighing, flushing, cramps, paresthesias, dryness of the mouth, vasovagal fainting, insomnia, increased frequency of micturation, diarrhea and anorexia. Although some of these symptoms may be indicative of organic cardiac disease in certain circumstances, they are also readily recognized as symptoms of an anxiety state.

Signs: The patient is often thin and of asthenic build. A distaste for physical activity and a rapid resting heart rate are usually present. Blood pressure may be increased if the patient is excited when examined, but persistent readily with exercise or when the patient stands up after lying down or squatting. Return of the heart to normal after exercise is delayed. Hyperventilation and tachypnea are common, particularly with stress, but no abnormal physical signs other than occasional systolic ejection murmurs are found on examination. The presence of hemodynamically insignificant organic heart disease, a trivial "functional" murmur, or insignificant electrocardiographic changes may complicate the picture and it may be extremely difficult to decide which problems are functional.

Differential Diagnosis

Active rheumatic fever, rheumatic carditis, anemia, thyrotoxicosis, systemic arteriovenous fistula, tuberculosis, pleurisy, influenza or any high output state must be differentiated from neurocirculatory asthenia. The diagnosis of effort syndrome probably includes more than one condition; with time, various different syndromes will probably be identified. There is almost certainly a relationship between effort syndrome and poor physical activity for the general population. Physical inactivity tends to produce a physiologic state resemblance that seen in effort syndrome. Prolonged bed rest, debilitating illness or simple inactivity all reduce exercise tolerance cause disproportionate tachycardia and result in marked tiredness after effort. Physical training programs are capable of altering the response to exercise. In Sweden, a group of patients identified as having "vasoregulatory asthenia" underwent a training program, which resulted in significant improvement in symptoms and exercise tolerance.

The physiologic "defect" in untrained persons is a failure in the mechanisms distributing cardiac output to different parts of the systemic circulation. Muscular exercise involves a marked increase in muscle blood flow. As a compensatory mechanism, perfusion of non-essential parts of the systemic circulation (skin, kidneys, other viscera and nonexercising muscles) is ordinarily reduced. If nonessential perfusion is maintained, the total cardiac output for a given work load is greater than normal; a higher pulse rate and limited exercises tolerance result. Training programs can reduce both cardiac output and heart rate at submaximal loads and increase the subject's maximal exercises performance. The arteriovenous oxygen difference at a given work load consequently increases. The statement that training increases the amount of oxygen extracted by the muscles is not correct. The arteriovenous oxygen difference is increased because a larger proportion of cardiac output perfuses the exercising muscles and blood draining exercising muscles is low in oxygen content.

ABNORMAL POSITION OF THE HEART

Cause of Abnormal Position of the Heart: Associated Conditions

Displacement of the heart interferes with physical examination more than it impairs function of the heart. Abnormalities on the ECG and chest X-ray due to displacement of the heart are also confusing and often suggest more serious abnormalities than are actually present. Abnormal position of the heart may be due to congenital abnormalities, as in dextrocardia, dextroversion or absence of the left pericardium. It may be due to lung disease, which either pushes or pulls the heart and mediastinal

contents to one side or to abnormalities of the thoracic cage, which may be congenital or acquired. There may be associated congenital abnormalities in the heart itself, especially when chest deformity is congenital. Chest deformity also occurs as a result of congenital heart disease. Cardiac deformity also occurs as a result of congenital heart disease. Cardiac hypertrophy in children with a soft cartilaginous thorax tends to produce a bulge in the left upper chest, which is seen well in ventricular septal defect. The developing thorax becomes fixed in its abnormal shape, and the deformity persists into adult life. The heart itself may be normally situated, but the great vessels may be abnormal, as in right-sided aortic arch or absence of the left pulmonary artery, which may occur as isolated lesions or with Fallot's tetralogy. A left sided superior vena cava and the inferior vena cava may enter the right atrium in an abnormal position. These lesions are seen with atrial septal defects but can also occur alone.

Dextrocardia and Dextroversion

The heart may be situated in the right side of the chest either because of mirror image dextrocardia or because of dextroversion. Dextrocardia is usually associated with complete situs inversus involving the abdominal viscera; it is also found with other congenital heart anomalies. In dextroversion, the cardiac chambers are on the correct side, but the heart is twisted and lies more to the right and more in the right side of the chest than normal. Dextroversion is also associated with congenital heart lesions. The position of the heart per se has no effect on its function.

Displacement Due to Lung Disease

The heart can be either pulled to one side by fibrosis of collapse of the ipsilateral lung or pushed by pleural effusion or pneumothorax to the contralateral side. The mediastinal contents are shifted as one unit, and the function of the heart is seldom if ever affected. The largest displacement is seen in patients who have undergone lung removal and bizarre radiologic findings appear when overdistention of the remaining lung leads to herniation of the lung to opposite side of the thorax.

Displacement Due to Abnormalities of the Thoracic Cage

Displacement of the heart due to pectus excavatum and kyphoscoliosis may cause physical findings suggestive of heart disease. Since associated congenital heart lesions are common, the diagnosis is often difficult. Depression of the sternum may be associated with abnormalities of the position of the thoracic spine. These abnormalities narrow the anteroposterior diameter of the thorax. In this case, the heart may appear enlarged on the posteroanterior view and narrowed on the lateral view. Systolic ejection murmurs, wide splitting of the second sound and even diastolic murmurs can occur. The ECG may also show an incomplete right bundle branch block and the large cardiac shadow on the posteroanterior view with a prominent right ventricular outflow tract may suggest atrial septal defect. In some cases, atrial septal defect is actually present. In kyphoscoliosis, the heart is often rotated, usually toward a right anterior oblique position. The outflow tract is thus abnormally prominent. The ECG shows clockwise rotation of the heart as a result of cardiac displacement and it is often difficult to be sure that the heart is normal. Patients with chest deformity not infrequently complain of symptoms similar to those of effort syndrome, e.g. dyspnea, palpitations, sweating, fatigue, noncardiac pain and nervousness. In the large majority of cases, there is no underlying heart disease and no specific cardiac treatment is indicated.

■ HEART DISEASE IN PREGNANCY

Introduction

What if a pregnant lady comes to you for cardiac evaluation?

Heart disease in pregnancy has become a less important clinical problem in the developed countries in recent years because valvular and congenital heart diseases are now recognized and treated prior to childbearing age. Rheumatic heart disease, especially mitral stenosis, accounts for about 90% of cases of heart disease in pregnant women but most of these women have mild valvular disease because those with more severe types have had surgical treatment. Acute rheumatic fever, the precursor of rheumatic valvular heart disease is much less common today than was the case 20–30 years ago, in part because of antibiotic (chronic penicillin or sulfonamide) prophylaxis against streptococcal infections and in part because of prompt treatment of streptococcal infection when they do occur. The prevalence in developing countries is difficult to determine but because cardiac surgery is less frequently performed in those countries, the clinical problems of management of pregnancy in women with severe mitral stenosis still arise.

Congenital heart disease is now recognized at a much earlier age as a result of greater availability of neonatal and pediatric cardiac care units. With the exception of the infrequent Eisenmeneger syndrome, in which shunt defects are associated with severe pulmonary hypertension, severe congenital heart disease is treated surgically before childbearing age. Awareness of the importance of rubella in the first trimester of pregnancy and its prevention by immunization before pregnancy occurs has resulted in a marked decrease in the incidence of rubella in early pregnancy, one of the common causes of congenital heart disease. The incidence of congenital heart disease has not decreased in recent years, but the frequency of the problem of untreated congenital heart disease in pregnancy is less now; even before the advent of open heart surgery, it was responsible for only 3–5% of all cases of heart disease in pregnancy.

Classification

Pregnant patients with heart disease can be distinguished into two general categories. The first category consists of women with pre-existing heart disease in whom the physiologic load imposed by pregnancy increases the work of the heart. In such cases, if the reserve capacity of the heart is compromised, the heart may fail.

The second category is made up of women with disease induced by pregnancy, e.g. Pre-eclampsia eclampsia, peripartum cardiopathy, thromboembolic disease causing multiple pulmonary emboli and pulmonary hypertension and dissection of aorta.

Pre-existing heart disease is usually valvular or congenital but other types must be recognized also. Hypertension, mitral valve prolapse and hypertrophic cardiomyopathy all may occur in women of childbearing age. Coronary heart disease is sufficiently rare at this age that it does not cause a clinical problem except in women with severe juvenile onset diabetes mellitus or homozygous genetic hypercholesterolemia. Coronary heart disease may appear in the 20s in these conditions.

Physiologic Changes in the Mother as a Result of Pregnancy

The most striking cardiovascular change in pregnancy is an increase in the cardiac output of about 30% by the third or fourth month, usually owing to increased stroke volume because the heart rate increases only slightly about 10 beats/min. Oxygen consumption increases to a lesser extent about 20%. Systemic vascular resistance decreases despite the raised cardiac output because of the arteriovenous fistula like pregnant placenta and possibly as a result of increased prostaglandin production. There is a marked increase in total body water of about 7 liters of which 75% is extracellular, reaching a maximum in the second trimester. Plasma volume and red cell volume also increase in normal pregnancy. The increased extracellular fluid is to only a slight extent the result of aldosterone secretion, which is but modestly raised in most pregnancies. Plasma rennin and angiotensin are increased, yet the blood pressure in most normal pregnancies not only does not

rise but actually falls, especially in the first and second trimesters. Body weight increases an average of about 10 kg.

The glomerular filtration rate increases up to 30–50% above normal during normal pregnancy, although it decreases in pre-eclampsia. This results in a greatly increased filtered in pre-eclampsia. This results in a greatly increased filtered load of sodium, all of which is reabsorbed or excreted except for a small amount, which is progressively retained, so that by the end of pregnancy approximately 500 mEq of sodium ate retained in the extracellular fluid volume and in the developing fetus. Tubular sodium reabsorption greatly exceeds the amount that can be attributed to aldosterone and the mechanism for the very large increase is not known. The role of progesterone has been studied because it increases at least 300 fold during pregnancy, antagonizes aldosterone and causes excretion of sodium in normal women, perhaps by decreasing renovascular resistance and thus rennin secretion. It undoubtedly influences blood volume changes of pregnancy.

The relative increase in plasma and blood volume in comparison to red cell mass accounts for the hemoglobin during pregnancy, which often is confused with true anemia.

Because the physiologic changes occur early in pregnancy by the beginning of the second trimester, patients with cardiac disease may develop symptoms of cardiac failure early in pregnancy if their cardiac reserve limited and in such cases intervention such as therapeutic abortion can be performed per vagina. The load of pregnancy continues throughout the entire period of gestation and some patients may tolerate pregnancy well until the last 1–2 months despite the fact that the load has been present all through pregnancy.

In the latter part of pregnancy, the position of the mother is quite important in influencing cardiac output which is reduced in the supine position (by mechanically obstructing the inferior vena cava and decreasing venous return) and increased in the lateral position.

Oxygen consumption at rest increases progressively during pregnancy whereas cardiac output increases in the first and second trimesters and for unknown reasons falls in the last several weeks of pregnancy. This discrepancy is due to the arteriovenous fistula like function of the placenta. The high output state resemblances that seen in arteriovenous fistulas and the patient has a hyperdynamic cardiac impulse, a raised venous pressure, dilated and pulsating digital arteries, a warm skin and decreased systemic vascular resistance. The importance of the uterine and placental blood flow has been emphasized. Impairment of perfusion of these organs may be important in the development of pre-eclampsia.

Physiologic Changes with Labor and the Puerperium

In addition to marked changes in arterial and pulse pressure and in pulse rate with uterine contractions during labor, cardiac output increases with each contraction, especially in the supine position.

Most of the hemodynamic changes return to normal by 10 days after delivery. With the exception of peripartum cardiomyopathy, cardiac complications of pregnancy are rare after the tenth day.

Cardiac Complications of Pregnancy

As indicated previously, the cardiovascular load of normal pregnancy is large, but most normal women and women with mild valvular or congenital heart disease or hypertension tolerate pregnancy without difficulty. If cardiac function is impaired in the prepregnant state (New York Heart Association class II or IV) or worsens in the few weeks of pregnancy, cardiac complication progressively increases. Patients who had cardiac failure in a previous pregnancy are more apt to develop cardiac failure in the current pregnancy.

The most serious varieties of heart disease complicating pregnancy are severe mitral or aortic stenosis, Eisenmenger's syndrome and severe coarctation of aorta, cardiac failure may be anticipated as pregnancy continues and may cause serious problems at the time of delivery.

Difficulty in Diagnosis of Heart Disease in Pregnancy

The recognition of cardiac disease or of early cardiac failure may be difficult in pregnant women, especially if they have not been seen prior to pregnancy. The increased blood volume, cardiac output and hyperdynamic cardiac state may cause cardiac ejection murmurs, raised venous pressure, hyperdynamic cardiac impulse, physiologic S_3, symptoms of dyspnea and especially later in pregnancy, edema resulting from sodium retention. These normal physiologic changes of pregnancy must be recognized as such and not attributed to cardiac disease or cardiac failure. Vital capacity does not normally change during pregnancy and a decrease indicated developing pulmonary venous congestion. A measurement of basal vital interpret changes; a single test is not valid.

Recognition of the underlying cardiac disease is based on the same cardinal clinical features that characterize the diagnosis in the nonpregnant state.

Hypertension in Pregnancy

The management of hypertension, whether from hypertensive disease of pregnancy (pre-eclampsia), pre-existing hypertension or the hypertension of coarctation is the most important because of the hazard of aortic dissection and cardiac failure in the presence of hypertension. It is estimated at least half of all cases of dissection of the aorta in women occur during pregnancy, not all of them in women with hypertension.

Hypertensive Disorders of Pregnancy

Hypertension during pregnancy may be independent of pregnancy, as occurs in essential hypertension, pheochromocytoma or coarctation of the aorta or it may be a complication of pregnancy such as occurs in pre-eclampsia. The latter two are collectively referred to in the older literature as toxemia of pregnancy. The differentiation between essential hypertension and toxemia of pregnancy with pre-eclampsia depends upon the period either precedes pregnancy when raised blood pressure occurs. In essential hypertension, raised arterial pressure either precedes pregnancy or occurs early in pregnancy, before the last trimester, whereas pre-eclampsia is characterized by a normal blood pressure prior to pregnancy or early in pregnancy but a rise in pressure in the last trimester. Pre-eclampsia may complicate essential hypertension in which case the blood pressure is raised early in pregnancy and later in pregnancy, the pressure increases substantially and is associated with proteinuria and edema. Pheochromocytoma and coarctation of the aorta are independent processes.

Essential Hypertension

If a measurement above 140 mm Hg systolic or 90 mm Hg diastolic on a single reading is considered to constitute hypertension as many as 20% of young women may have elevated pressures. There is no sharp division between normal blood pressure and hypertension and liability of pressure is characteristic of all individuals whether they are normal or hypertensive. The problem is complicated in pregnant women because vasodilation produces a fall in pressure in the second trimester, perhaps as a result of the increased production of prostaglandins or other peptides. The magnitude of the fall can be significant, so that individual is needed hypertensive. The diagnosis of essential hypertension must be made almost exclusively on the basis if the arterial pressure itself, because in the age range of the usual pregnant patient, vascular complications are uncommon unless the hypertension is severe and the ECG and examination of the ocular fundi and heart usually show no abnormalities. If the hypertension is severe and if vascular complications such as fundal abnormalities, cardiac enlargement, left ventricular hypertrophy or impairment of renal function are present during the first few months of pregnancy, the likelihood of a significant rise of pressure in the last trimester, with the development of pre-eclampsia and an increased probability of fetal death, may indicate the need for therapeutic abortion.

Pre-eclampsia Eclampsia

The term toxemia of pregnancy is in a sense obsolete, since no toxins have been discovered to produce the clinical syndrome of hypertension, edema and proteinuria, developing in the last trimester of pregnancy is a continuum progressing at various rates and extending from the mildest forms of pre-eclampsia to severe eclampsia with multiple severe convulsions. Pre-eclampsia occurs in about 5% of all pregnancies if one includes toxemia associated with hypertension. The figure is higher-up to 10% if toxemia with pyelonephritis is added, but the disorder has gradually declined in incidence in the past several decades (see Prognosis), possibly as a consequence of better prenatal care. Eclampsia is much less frequent, occurring in about 0.1% of pregnant women.

Etiology

The cause of pre-eclampsia is unknown and many theories have been offered without universal acceptance even though the condition had been extensively studied for many years. Certain facts are clear, however. The condition is more frequent in the first pregnancy, in patients with pre-existing hypertension, in twin pregnancies, in patients with a history of pre-eclampsia, in patients with hydatidiform mole, and in some population of black women. One theory offered is that pre-eclampsia results from impaired uteroplacental perfusion; this is supported by the observation that during pre-eclampsia, plasma volume, glomerular filtration rate and uterine and placental blood flow decreases about 25% in recumbency. The Gravid uterus has a poorer arterial blood supply in pre-eclampsia as compared to the abundant blood supply from the uterine, ovarian and other arteries.

Clinical Findings

Pre-eclampsia is defined as a syndrome encountered in the second half of pregnancy characterized by at least 2 of 3 cardinal manifestations.

1. A rather abrupt increase of blood pressure amounting to 30 mm or more systolic and 15 mm or more diastolic after the 26th week of pregnancy.
2. The appearance (or sudden increase) of proteinuria of at least 0.5 g/day.
3. Edema in the upper half of the body.

Any two of these must be manifest on two occasions at least 6 hours apart. If convulsions occur in addition to the above criteria, the case is classified as eclampsia.

Generalized edema is common in pregnancy and when present in the lower half of the body is not considered diagnosis of heart failure. The increased tubular reabsorption of sodium and water causes edema in the upper half of the body that may precede the appearance of proteinuria and hypertension. The progression of pre-eclampsia to eclampsia is an ominous development and approximately 5–10% of patients with eclampsia die of the disease.

Apart from the clinical manifestation of weight gain, edema in the upper half of the body, proteinuria, and hypertension, patients with pre-eclampsia may develop headache, drowsiness, visual disturbances, dyspnea and if the hypertension is severe, pulmonary edema and cardiac failure. Cerebral hemorrhage is the cause of death in about 10% of patients with eclampsia who die. Acute tubular necrosis is an uncommon cause of death but may occur in severe toxemia. Hypotension may develop because of adrenocortical insufficiency.

Clinical Course

The onset of pre-eclampsia may be gradual or sudden and the diagnosis may be difficult to establish in the early stages. Patients may develop edema of a normal pregnancy. The proteinuria may be slight and variable. Any one of these findings should may be sufficient to reverse the process by increasing uterine, renal, and placental blood flow, but if proteinuria increases or if the blood pressure rises and especially if the patient develops symptoms such as blurred vision, decreased urine output or a rapid gain in weight, the patient should be considered to have pre-eclampsia and should be hospitalized. Examination of the ocular fundi is often helpful; a "shimmering edema" of the retina is said to be characteristics of pre-eclampsia, but this findings has not been universally accepted. Papilledema, hemorrhages and exudates are rare but may occur. The development of a generalized boring headache is the most reliable symptom of an impending convulsion and should be the immediate indication for more intensive hospital therapy, including termination of pregnancy.

Chapter 10

Thyrotoxic Heart Disease and Some other Heart Diseases of Clinical Importance

■ INTRODUCTION

One can suspect the diagnosis by noting the warm, moist hands and relatively quick movements, which are surprising for a patient in heart failure. There is often a disparity between the vigor of the patient and the symptoms and signs of heart failure.

Overlooked thyrotoxicosis: Thyrotoxicosis should always be suspected in patients with unexplained atrial fibrillation or congestive heart failure poorly responsive to digitalis therapy or inpatients with systolic hypertension with a wide pulse pressure and a normal or short circulation time. This latter finding is in contrast to the delayed circulation time usually seen in patients with cardiac failure.

Absence of thyrotoxic symptoms: In so-called apathetic thyrotoxicosis, the patient is subdued and lacking in energy instead of excited and nervous. There is, however, a disparity between the apathetic facies and hyperactive movements noted on alert examination. It is often helpful to compare the apparent well being of the patient with the severity of symptoms. Patients with apathetic facies may have tremor, but hyperactive movements are more common. Increased peripheral blood flow with hyperemia often results in what has been called "salmon skin", which is a helpful clinical feature.

Cardiac symptoms and signs: Cardiac manifestations may precede obvious evidence of thyrotoxicosis such signs, mainly atrial fibrillation, may precede the other clinical signs of thyrotoxicosis by months or years. Careful observation and repeated studies for thyroid disease may permit recognition of the development of thyrotoxic heart disease when it was not obvious at the onset of atrial fibrillation.

Differential Diagnosis

Overt thyrotoxicosis is usually so obvious that few diseases should be confused with it. When the clinical picture is incomplete, especially in early cases, the diagnosis can be confusing. Anxiety is one of the most important conditions to be distinguished because of the nervousness, tremor, tachycardia, sweating and similar symptoms that occur in that state. Evidence of a raised cardiac output, including vasodilatation and warm, moist skin, is important in differentiating thyrotoxic patients from those with anxiety states, in whom there may be increased sweating but a cold and moist skin. Other manifestations of hyperthyroidism, such as unexplained weight loss and diarrhea, may be helpful diagnostic clues. Sleeping tachycardia is an important sign. Other causes of unexplained atrial fibrillation must be excluded if this is the presenting symptom or sign (e.g. "silent" mitral stenosis, atrial septal defect, coronary heart disease, left atrial myxoma, infective endocarditis). If weakness and weight loss are the dominant findings one must exclude neoplasms, various types of myopathies, liver disease, myasthenia, and depression. If cardiac failure due to no apparent cause is the presenting manifestation, one must exclude ischemic coronary cardiomyopathy, or cardiomyopathy associated with various systemic disorders as well as common varieties of cardiac failure that may have obscure features (valvular heart disease, atrial septal defect, "burned out" hypertension, coronary disease, and cardiac failure resulting from untreated atrial fibrillation with a rapid ventricular rate).

Definitive diagnosis in these atypical cases is possible with the use of relatively specific biochemical studies, notably serum T3, T4 and if necessary radioiodine uptake. These tests may be interfered with by previous iodine intake, either as medication or during radiologic studies using iodine-containing contrast media.

MYXEDEMA AND MYXEDEMA HEART

Myxedema heart is a well-known entity described to be associated with cardiac failure because two-thirds of patients with myxedema may have enlargement of the cardiac silhouette as shown by radiology. More recent physiologic studies have shown that in most myxedema patients pericardial effusion and not cardiac failure is responsible for the enlarged cardiac shadow seen radiologically. Investigations using echocardiography have shown that some patients have dilatation of the left ventricle without significant pericardial effusion with an essentially normal cardiac shadow, while a third group have a combination of cardiac dilation and pericardial effusion. The cardiac shadow may be enlarged even after all pericardial fluid has been removed. The cause of the effusion is not clearly understood.

In one large series of cases of myxedema, the disease occurred spontaneously in 40% of patients, but in the remaining 60% it followed either I therapy or thyroidectomy. At present, many more cases of myxedema are seen following successful I therapy, and it is feared that with the passage of time the numbers will increase. When a patient with thyrotoxicosis improves following administration of radio iodine, the physician must continue to be alert for the late appearance of myxedema.

Clinical Findings

Symptoms

The symptoms of myxedema include weakness, fatigue, dry and puffy skin, hoarseness, thick tongue, and slow pulse. Patients with myxedema heart characteristically complain of exertional fatigue more than dyspnea, angina due to associated coronary disease, and periorbital and peripheral edema. The pulse volume has a small amplitude, with a weak carotid upstroke in contrast to what would be expected in bradycardia.

Two uncommon symptoms are perhaps not fully appreciated. One is the frequency of paresthesia and perceptive deafness, which occurred in about half of cases in Wayne's series. Another symptom frequently helpful in diagnosis is husky hoarseness. On more than one occasion, myxedema has been strongly suspected in a patient with heart disease entirely on the basis of voice. Coarse dry skin changes may also be obvious as helpful in diagnosis.

That the cardiac manifestations of myxedema are usually due to pericardial effusion rather than cardiac failure is supported by the rarity of clinical congestive failure and the frequency of effusion as shown on echocardiography. Physical signs such as orthopnea, raised venous pressure usually absent, and, despite an abrupt increase in the size of the heart shadow, pulmonary venous congestion is often absent. Following the removal of pericardial fluid, the cardiac size is usually (not always) found to be normal.

The cardiac border may appear to be enlarged but the weak and distant heart sounds and the difficulty in palpating the apical impulse make an accurate clinical determination of heart size difficult and should make one suspect hypothyroidism.

The slow pulse may be only relative in patients with myxedema. For example, the heart rate may be only 60–70 beats/min, which would be an unusual findings in a patient with cardiomegaly and presumes congestive heart failure.

Patients may have effusions in the pericardial, pleural and peritoneal cavities because of the slow development of effusion large amounts of pericardial fluid may be found (2000–4000 mL).

Differential Diagnosis

The diagnosis of myxedema is frequently missed because the clinical manifestations occur slowly and subtly and may be attributed to aging, i.e. as the patient tires more easily and becomes slower in through and movement. Many patients with a diagnosis of myxedema are treated initially for anemia. Periorbital nonpitting edema, generalized collections of serous fluid, and proteinuria may suggest nephritis. Finally, the diagnosis of cardiomyopathy is often made in myxedematous patients because of the presence of presumed cardiomegaly on radiologic examination.

There may be a delay of 5-10 years between the onset of symptoms and the diagnosis of myxedema.

Alcoholic Cardiomyopathy

This is a subject of some controversy because alcohol may produce cardiomyopathy by a primary toxic effect on the heart, by nutritional deficiency (especially of thiamine, as in beriberi heart disease) if the individual does not eat an adequate diet, or as a result of additives (cobalt in cobalt-beet cardiomyopathy). Chronic alcoholics may have intermittent thiamine deficiency or excessive requirements for thiamine, as when they develop fever from infections, or after a high-carbohydrate diet; therefore, a mixed picture of toxic alcoholic cardiomyopathy and nutritional beriberi heart disease may be found.

There is no clear-cut boundary between cardiovascular beriberi and non-thiamine-responsive myocardial disease. Dietary deficiency of protein or calories infrequently causes chronic congestive cardiomyopathy (which is more frequently due to alcohol) and should be differentiated from it. In populations, afflicted by famine and in prisoners of war examined after a weight loss of about 20 kg, cardiac enlargement, hypoproteinemia, and cardiac failure are rarely seen; cardiac atrophy is much more common. Endomyocardial fibrosis has been thought by some to be related to inadequate nutrition.

Involvement of the Liver

Alcohol not only affects the cells of the myocardium by direct toxic action; it also affects the cells of the liver, even in patients receiving good diets with adequate vitamins. As a result, patients may present with hepatic involvement as well as cardiac disease, although some patients are above to drink large amounts of alcohol for many years without developing either cardiac or hepatic disease, or one but not the other.

Relationship of Beriberi Heart Disease to Alcoholic Cardiomyopathy

Beriberi heart disease, when clearly related to thiamine deficiency, was described by Wenckebach in 1929 (Wenckebach, 1934) and by Soma Weiss in 1937. High output failure is the dominant clinical feature in most cases, but some had low cardiac output because of delay in treatment. In contrast to the hyperkinetic circulation with tachycardia, raised cardiac output, and warm extremities of patients with beriberi heart disease, the patient with alcoholic cardiomyopathy has signs of low cardiac output, relatively weak pulses of small volume, and cold extremities. The heart is large and bulky, with a markedly decreased ejection fraction. Large doses of thiamine are ineffective in treatment of alcoholic cardiomyopathy, in contrast to beriberi heart disease, but a hyperkinetic circulation (overactive, high cardiac output) can be produced in a week in a chronic alcoholic who develops a fever or abruptly reduced thiamine intake.

Beriberi heart was formerly common in developing countries and found occasionally in the USA before recognition of the need for thiamine replacement and the ready availability of vitamin supplements in patient receiving deficient diets. Alcoholic cardiomyopathy, however is common where large amounts of alcohol are consumed daily even with adequate nutrition and vitamins. In alcoholic cardiomyopathy with good nutrition (including vitamin supplements), left ventricular dysfunction can often be demonstrated by sophisticated techniques before the patient develops clinical symptoms or obvious signs of cardiac enlargement or failure. Most cases of alcoholic cardiomyopathy are probably due to a direct toxic action of alcohol on the myocardium.

Clinical Findings

The criteria for the cardiac diagnosis of alcoholic cardiomyopathy are similar to those of idiopathic cardiomyopathy or chronic congestive cardiomyopathy, with the exception of the history of alcoholic intake. The typical clinical picture is idiopathic cardiac failure in a man in the early middle years without coronary heart disease, hypertension, valvular heart disease or congenital heart disease. There is no history of valvular or congenital heart disease but a definite history of large alcohol intake over a period of many years; most patients have drunk more than 250 mL of whiskey or its equivalent every day for at least 10 years. Brigden (1964) has emphasized the importance of alcohol in chronic idiopathic heart disease and believes that it is responsible for at least half of all cases of chronic congestive cardiomyopathy.

A. Symptoms: The onset is usually insidious, with nonspecific fatigue, dyspnea, palpitations and possibly edema.

B. Sign: there may be cardiac enlargement and evidences of left ventricular failure. When cardiac failure develops, it is low output failure, and the patient usually has all the clinical features of that condition. The cardiac failure is chiefly left ventricular, but there may be right ventricular failure as well, with raised venous pressure, tricuspid insufficiency, and a rapid small pulse. There is usually a left or right ventricular heave, gallop rhythm, murmurs of functional mitral or tricuspid insufficiency and pulmonary rates, enlarged tender liver, and dependent edema. Although the arterial blood pressure may be elevated during the phase of severe failure with compensatory systemic vasoconstriction, the pressure falls to normal when failure is improved with routine cardiac therapy.

Differential Diagnosis

Alcoholic cardiomyopathy must be distinguished from other disorders that produce congestive cardiomyopathy in patients with long histories of excessive alcohol intake. Hypertension is excluded by normal blood pressure after restoration to the compensated state; coronary artery disease by the absence of angina pectoris or myocardial infarction clinically or electrocardiographically and, if necessary, by negative coronary angiogram; valvular heart disease by the absence of a history, of murmurs and by decrease of murmurs when compensation is restored. Congenital heart disease is excluded by a negative history and no abnormalities of congenital heart disease on cineangiograms, and echocardiography.

Chapter 11

Cardiac Arrhythmias

■ INTRODUCTION

Sometimes it is essential to diagnose cardiac arrhythmias clinically without aid of sophisticated investigations. Tachy and brady arrhythmias are equally important.

Clinical Features of Tachyarrhythmias in General

A. Palpitations: Palpitations, which are subjective sensations of the patient, may be due to increased forcefulness of the heartbeat as well as to arrhythmia. Furthermore, a disturbance in rhythm may be intermittent and on one occasion be due to arrhythmia and on another to a forceful heartbeat. Therefore, arrhythmia must be documented by continuous ambulatory electrocardiographic monitoring to distinguish the cause of palpitations.

B. Initial Assessment of the Nature of the Arrhythmia and Its Impact on the Patient: The approach to the patient with a cardiac arrhythmia requires first an assessment of the precise diagnosis of the arrhythmia and an estimate of its severity (i.e., the impact of the arrhythmia on left ventricular function, blood pressure, cerebral and coronary perfusion, and renal function). The importance of the heart rate, the duration of the arrhythmia, and the presence of underlying heart rate, the duration of the arrhythmia, and the presence of underlying heart disease must be reemphasized. As stated in the general introduction, the arrhythmia may be trivial or urgent depending upon the age of the patient, the cause of the arrhythmia, and the effect of the arrhythmia on the circulation. The disturbance in rhythm may be intermittent, and its presence must be documented by continuous ambulatory electrocardiographic monitoring in doubtful cases because palpitations may be due to increased forcefulness of the heartbeat and not to arrhythmia.

C. Variable Difficulty of Diagnosis: The diagnosis may be simple—at the bedside or after a routine ECG—or it may be very complex, requiring extensive studies with carotid sinus massage, Valsalva's maneuver, rapid atrial pacing. His bundle studies with intracardiac recording and stimulation, and in selected cases, coronary arteriography and left ventricular cineangiograms to rule out cardiac aneurysm. It may be necessary to determine the relationship of the QRS complex and the P wave to the His bundle deflection, the effect of posture and drugs, and the adequacy of the baroreceptor reflexes in order to identify the type of arrhythmia and determine whether it is ventricular or supraventricular. The arrhythmia may be intermittent or short-lived. The relationship of the P waves to the QRS complexes requires careful study. A long ECG strip with each P wave and QRS complex identified is essential in the study of antegrade and retrograde conduction. Conduction delays or blocks may occur in limitless combinations and in both directions. New depolarizations in various parts of the heart, intermittent conduction with entrance and exit block to an ectopic focus (as in parasystole), and multiple arrhythmias may follow each other in rapid sequence. This is particularly true in acute myocardial infarction, in which, over a period of an hour, the patient may have multiple arrhythmias combined with conduction defects anywhere in the specialized conduction system. In most instances, however, careful consideration of the electrocardiographic evidence will allow the diagnosis to be made without the need for invasive procedures.

D. **Previous Attacks:** In assessing the importance of any given episode of arrhythmia, the examiner should obtain a history of previous episodes, an indication of the patient's tolerance for them, their frequency and duration, the extent of circulatory impairment, and the response to treatment if any. Some arrhythmias last seconds or minutes, while others, such as atrial fibrillation, last hours or days or indefinitely. The examiner should keep separate the clinical features and treatment of an acute episode from measures taken to prevent a recurrent attack.

Symptoms

1. **Identification of arrhythmia:** The patient may have no symptoms at all, and the arrhythmia may be discovered on routine examination, in which the patient is found to have premature beats, atrial fibrillation or flutter or even ventricular tachycardia or transient brief episodes of ventricular fibrillation. Ambulatory electrocardiographic monitoring or graded exercise stress tests may precipitate both simple and complex arrhythmias when they are not seen on a routine ECG. Many patients with mitral stenosis have short bouts of atrial fibrillation without being aware of it. On the other hand, the onset of atrial fibrillation may be devastating, producing acute dyspnea, pulmonary edema, and an abrupt worsening of the clinical and hemodynamic state because of the inability to empty the left atrium and fill the left ventricle during the short diastolic pauses that are due to the rapid ventricular rate and the loss of atrial systole and dilatation of the left atrium. The usual history is of a sudden onset of palpitations that the patient may describe as regular or irregular, although it may not always be possible to characterize them one way or the other. It may help if the physician taps out various rhythms and rates and asks, "Is it like this?" etc. The patient may not complain of palpitations but rather of the consequences of the arrhythmia, such as weakness, chest pain, dizziness, dyspnea, and confusion. In paroxysmal atrial tachycardia, the patients may pass a large quantity of urine within a few minutes of onset a phenomenon that is thought to be due to inhibition of vasopressin secretion by the posterior pituitary, although the hypothesis has not been proved. The mechanism by which this occurs is not known. LA might be involved. Hemodynamic studies in paroxysmal atrial tachycardia may in some cases show not only a marked increase in heart rate but also prolongation of the P-R interval, fall in arterial pressure, decrease in the cardiac index, and increase in the pulmonary artery diastolic pressure and right atrial pressure.

2. **Progressive deterioration of cardiac function:** The symptoms of an arrhythmia may not be apparent at the onset. In arrhythmias of longer duration, there may be progressive deterioration of cardiac function, with impaired perfusion of vital organs from decreased cardiac output. The patient may then develop symptoms resulting from inadequate perfusion of the brain, heart, kidneys, skin and extremities. The fact that the patient tolerates the arrhythmia at the

outset does not guarantee that circulatory embarrassment will not develop with time. This is especially true in patients in the coronary care unit, in whom cardiac failure may develop gradually.

Features of Special Importance

The pause that follows the premature beat may allow the physician to diagnose the underlying cardiac condition, and it is useful to listen carefully to the postpause beat. In aortic stenosis, for example, the murmur may be louder as a result of the more forceful ventricular contraction following the pause. However, this is not the case in mitral regurgitation. The long pause with increase left ventricular volume may produce or increase left ventricular outflow obstruction in hypertrophic cardiomyopathy and the first sound may be diminished in the postpause beat. When long pauses are felt at the wrist or at the carotid arteries, the possibility of a "dropped" beat due to atrioventricular block must be considered. Even early premature beats can be heard with the stethoscope (unless they are non-conducted atrial premature beats) whereas during "dropped" beats there is no ventricular sound.

Diagnosis

Supraventricular tachycardia is recognized by a sudden increase in heart rate to 150–250/min, although rates of 300/min. have been observed in infants, probably because atrioventricular conduction is accelerated in infants and the refractory period of the atrioventricular node is shorter. It is regular.

Diagnostic Features of Paroxysmal Atrial Tachycardia

A. **Degree of Atrioventricular Conduction**: Conduction is usually 1:1, and there is no clinical evidence of atrial and ventricular asynchrony, so that there is nothing abnormal to be heard at the bedside other than the rapid heart rate. The first sound does not vary in intensity, and no cannon waves can be seen in the jugular venous pulse. The major exception occurs when the atrial tachycardia is due to digitalis toxicity, in which instance, because digitalis also decreases conduction through the atrioventricular node, 2:1 block is frequent and may be overlooked when the atrial rate is about 150/min and the ventricular rate about 75/min. As the ventricular rate is normal, the patient has no palpitations or other symptoms, and were it not for the evidence on the ECG of rapid atrial rates with 2:1 ventricular response, digitalis toxicity could be overlooked. Although digitalis is the usual cause of atrial tachycardia with 2:1 conduction, there are well-documented instances in which the patient has not received digitalis; the physician is thus not warranted in diagnosing digitalis toxicity on the basis of the arrhythmia alone.

Digitalis toxicity is less commonly manifested by atrial tachycardia with 1:1 conduction but may also produce partial progressive atrioventricular block with Wenckebach phenomenon.

B. **Jugular Venous Pulse:** It is helpful to study the jugular venous pulse carefully in these instances; rapid a waves at twice the rate of the ventricular response may lead to the correct diagnosis. The same is true in atrial flutter, when the conduction from the atria to the ventricular is 4:1 and the ventricular rate at 75/min. does not make one suspect that the atrial are.

Differential Diagnosis

In sinus tachycardia, the rate is rapid, essentially regular at short intervals, and usually less than 180/min. It may be slightly irregular and vary with simple maneuvers such as posture, mild exercise, respiration, breath holding, or carotid sinus pressure. The regularity of the heart rate in paroxysmal atrial tachycardia may differentiate this rhythm from sinus tachycardia, in which the heart rate may be rapid and apparently regular but can be altered by position, respiration, or slight exercise. If the heart rate is counted for a full minute, especially after changes in position and other maneuvers mentioned in the preceding sentence, it will be shown to be slightly irregular and variable in sinus tachycardia. In paroxysmal atrial tachycardia, however, the heart rate is not influenced by these procedures unless the attack is terminated abruptly. In ventricular tachycardia, careful inspection of the ECG or careful counting of the heart rate for 1 minute will show that the ventricular rate is often slightly irregular.

It is wise to count the heart rate for a full minute at intervals because in sinus tachycardia the rate will change, whereas in paroxysmal atrial or junctional tachycardia, it is usually regular and uninfluenced unless the attack is terminated abruptly.

Sinus tachycardia also has a background of one of a number of causative factors, e.g. fever, infection, anemia, anxiety, leukemia, thyrotoxicosis, or connective tissue disorders.

Clinical Differentiation

Clinical bedside evaluation may be valuable to provide evidence of atrial and ventricular asynchrony, e.g. varying intensity of the first heart sound and cannon waves in the jugular venous pulse. The signs of atrioventricular asynchrony may occur in His bundle or junctional tachycardia with atrioventricular dissociation, but this is uncommon. Cannon waves are large abrupt a waves in the jugular venous pulse ("venous Corrigan waves") occurring as the atria contract when the tricuspid valve is closed. They are often seen best when the patient is sitting and can be important clinical evidence, suggesting ventricular tachycardia when the ECG is doubtful.

Value of Underlying Condition in Differentiation: The age of the patient and the setting in which the tachycardia occurs are helpful in diagnosis. Ventricular tachycardia is more likely if the patient has acute myocardial infarction, coronary heart disease, or other disease of the left ventricle, such as hypertrophic cardiomyopathy, aortic stenosis, or hypertensive disease. As noted previously, if the patient is young and free of heart disease and the precipitating factor was an acute emotional event, supraventricular tachycardia is the more likely diagnosis. It must be emphasized again, however, that none of these criteria are absolute and all indicate only the probable site of origin of the tachycardia have no known or obvious heart disease, whereas supraventricular tachycardia may occur in patients with known heart disease even if the patient is young, so that one cannot rely exclusively on the age and underlying cardiac disease criteria. If it is essential to make the differentiation in order to determine therapy, His bundle recordings are helpful by demonstrating the presence of a His bundle spike preceding the QRS complex, in which case the tachycardia is supraventricular. His bundle recordings with intracardiac stimulation by programmed, critically timed supraventricular premature beats may establish the supraventricular origin of a tachycardia of unknown cause, but such procedures are indicated only if therapy is ineffective and the prognosis doubtful. In troublesome cases treatment should be directed towards the more serious condition, ventricular tachycardia; lidocaine with or without DC electric shock is helpful in both supraventricular and ventricular tachycardia.

ATRIAL FIBRILLATION AND ATRIAL FLUTTER

Atrial fibrillation is the most common atrial arrhythmia in older people. It can be paroxysmal or established, as is true of atrial flutter. Paroxysmal attacks usually last hours or days rather than seconds or minutes and almost never longer than 2 or 3 weeks. If the rhythm persists after this period, atrial fibrillation is said to be established, or chronic; this is in contrast to supraventricular tachycardia, which rarely lasts days or weeks and usually lasts minutes or hours. Paroxysmal atrial fibrillation may occur without known heart disease or other obvious reason but most commonly occurs after pulmonary or cardiac surgery or in older individuals with mitral stenosis, atrial septal defect, myocarditis, thyrotoxicosis, or constrictive pericarditis. It is most common in older people with left atrial enlargement due to any cause. It may be precipitated by an acute emotional event even if the patient has underlying cardiac disease such as mitral stenosis. It is not especially common in chronic coronary heart disease and is infrequent in acute myocardial infarction, although continuous monitoring has shown that it may occur. It is common when hypoxia and infection occur in chronic lung disease with cor pulmonale. Following pulmonary surgery—perhaps as a result of hypoxia from inadequate ventilation or pericardial injury—as many as one-third of patients may develop paroxysmal atrial fibrillation. Transient atrial fibrillation is also common following cardiac surgery, especially mitral valve surgery. Even if the rhythm reverts to sinus rhythm preoperatively, it often recurs after surgery. It is common during the course of untreated thyrotoxicosis and usually disappears spontaneously when the thyrotoxicosis is treated. It may be precipitated by cardiac catheterization in patients with mitral stenosis or atrial septal defect. For reasons that are not clear, atrial fibrillation is infrequent prior to infective endocarditis. It is common after the endocarditis is established in aortic or mitral valvular heart disease but uncommon in acute endocarditis in drug users with tricuspid and aortic valve lesions. Although it has been stated that coarse fibrillation (prominent fibrillation waves) is more common in rheumatic heart disease, we believe this differentiation is unreliable and too variable to depend on.

Atrial fibrillation is rare in pure aortic valve disease in the absence of failure, and its presence should prompt the physician to think of associated mitral valve disease even if the typical murmurs are not readily heard.

Clinical Course

The onset of atrial fibrillation may produce immediate symptoms of dyspnea in the patient with mitral stenosis and may also produce cardiac failure in the patient with atrial septal defect, when the rapid ventricular rate prevents atrial emptying and left ventricular filling. In mitral stenosis, left atrial pressure may rise quickly, producing pulmonary venous congestion, severe dyspnea and acute pulmonary edema. The atrial transport function of atrial systole may be required to preserve adequate left ventricular filling in patients with low cardiac reserve; the onset of atrial fibrillation may produce severe left ventricular failure in these patient. Some individuals merely have palpitations; a few may have no symptoms whatever, and the atrial fibrillation in these cases is discovered accidentally.

Atrial Fibrillation in Mitral Stenosis

Even when the ventricular rate at rest is controlled with digitalis, the onset of atrial fibrillation may convert an asymptomatic patient with moderate or severe mitral stenosis to a cardiac invalid because of the disproportionate rise in ventricular rate that occurs as atrioventricular conduction improves with exercise. The increased ventricular rate with exercise decreases left ventricular filling, raises left atrial pressure, and produces pulmonary venous congestion. Individuals who are totally asymptomatic, with normal pulmonary capillary wedge pressures during sinus rhythm, may have marked symptoms and a considerably rise in pulmonary capillary wedge pressure when they develop atrial fibrillation. Patients with mitral stenosis who have similar ventricular rates at rest when they are in sinus rhythm or atrial fibrillation with a controlled ventricular rate may have a considerable rise in ventricular rate even with mild exercise when in atrial fibrillation. Mild exercise may produce a ventricular rate of 90/min when the patient is in sinus rhythm and 120–130/min when the rhythm is atrial fibrillation.

The manner in which the patient with mitral stenosis handles atrial fibrillation, is a clue to the severity of the lesion; if the patient merely has palpitations and a sense of irregularity of heart rate without significant dyspnea, it can be inferred that the mitral stenosis is trivial.

Chronic Atrial Fibrillation

In chronic atrial fibrillation, especially if the ventricular rate is controlled with digitalis, the patient may be asymptomatic and may be unaware of the atrial fibrillation or its irregularity except when exercising. Some patients described what they think are paroxysmal episodes of atrial fibrillation when in fact they have chronic fibrillation but are aware of the rapid, irregular ventricular rate only with exercise or emotion.

Pulse Deficit

Before treatment is given, there is a substantial difference in ventricular rate as determined at the apex of the heart and that, which is felt at the radial pulse, the so-called pulse deficit. This occurs because the more rapid beats may not result in a sufficient stroke output to cause a pulse wave to reach the wrist. Following digitalis therapy, when the ventricular rate is slowed, each beat has a more forceful output and the pulse deficit diminishes. If the apical and radial rates are plotted before and during digitalis therapy, the disappearance or decrease of the pulse deficit is often a good index of adequate therapy.

Clinical Findings

Patients may be asymptomatic or may complain of a forceful heartbeat that follows the extra-systolic pause. In contrast to atrial premature beats, when there is a normal sequence of conduction via the atrioventricular node through to the ventricles, ventricular premature beats by retrograde activation depolarize the atrioventricular node and interrupt the normal sequence.

A. **Cannon Waves:** Right atrial systole may find the tricuspid valve closed because of recent intermittent ectopic ventricular systoles and produce, irregularly, a cannon wave in the neck as atrial systole forces blood back into the jugular vein, cannon waves are presystolic, of relatively large amplitude, and have a rapid ascent and descent, which has suggested the term "venous Corrigan" waves. The ventricular premature contractions occur irregularly; the sinus P wave and the ectopic QRS complexes may occur relatively simultaneously, usually with the P wave following the QRS complex, so that atrial contraction finds the triauspid valve closed. Occasionally, there may be 1:1 synchronous retrograde conduction to the sinus node with ventricular premature beats, and cannon waves do not occur, as is true also if the patient has atrial fibrillation or atrial flutter with significant or absent atrial systole.

B. **Evidence of Asynchrony of Atria and Ventricles:** The first heart sound may vary in intensity because of the asynchronous contraction of the atria and the ventricles, just as a complete atrioventricular block. The basic rate of sinus rhythm is not altered with ventricular premature beats. If the ventricular premature beats are frequent or occur in irregular runs, the cardiac rhythm may be so irregular that it may be confused with atrial fibrillation. Cannon waves in the neck may be helpful in the differentiation, as may the recognition of the "quick" premature beat before each pause.

Clinical Findings in Ventricular Tachycardia

Ventricular tachycardia should be strongly suspected when an abrupt tachycardia occurs in an older patient with coronary heart disease, especially if the patient had ventricular premature beats before the tachycardia and the QRS complexes are wide and bizarre, with QR or QS complexes in lead V_1, or if the complexes are similar to those seen in the ventricular premature beats present on a prior occasion. The T wave is usually large and in the direction opposite to that of the QRS complex.

A. **Differentiation from Supraventricular or Junctional Tachycardia with Aberrant Conduction**: Prolongation of the QRS complex and atrioventricular dissociation are not absolute criteria to establish the ventricular origin of a tachycardia.

B. **Asynchrony or Atrial and Ventricular Contractions:** The most important clinical features of ventricular tachycardia are asynchrony of atrial and ventricular contractions, with the atria beating at a slower rate. This is not an absolute criterion because independence of atrial and ventricular activity is occasionally due to junctional atrioventricular rhythms with retrograde atrioventricular block causing atrioventricular dissociation. Further, it must be remembered that retrograde activation of the atria may occur in ventricular tachycardia with a one-to-one conduction, so that asynchronous atrial and ventricular activity do not occur.

On auscultation because of the wide QRS complexes and atrioventricular dissociation, there is wide splitting of the first and second heart sounds, beat-to-beat variation in arterial pressures and systolic murmurs, changing intensity of the first heart sound depending upon the relation of the P wave to the QRS complex, and intermittent, large cannon a waves in the jugular venous pulse. When the relationship between atrial and ventricular contraction is such that the mitral and tricuspid valves are wide open at the onset of ventricular systole, they close with a snap and the first heart sound is louder. When the atria and the ventricle contract close together, the mitral valve leaflets are relatively closed and the first sound is soft. The systolic blood pressure varies from beat to beat depending upon the sequence of the atrial and ventricular contraction and the contribution of atrial systole to ventricular filling. If ventricular excitation is transmitted backward to the atrium or sinus node, the result is 1:1 ventriculoatrial conduction with no variation in the intensity of the first heart sound and no cannon waves in the jugular venous pulse.

Chapter 12

Frequently Asked Questions (FAQs) in Bedside Clinical Examination and Viva Voce

Here is an assortment of certain questions likely to be asked in one way or the other during practical examinations and during day to day clinical rounds. The main intention of this "mental gym" exercise is to sharpen your attitude towards common clinical problem solving and how to give "to the point" answers, which are liked by most of the examiners. The questions are endless but prototype questions of each topic may at times be very hardy for already overburdened UGs and PGs.

HISTORY TAKING

☐ If a patient comes to you with chest pain, how can you be reasonably sure clinically about the cause being ischemic cardiac pains or a local cause?
Answer: If patient comes with fist clenched in front of center of chest and is very vague about localization of pain, it is quite likely to be myocardial ischemica/infarct, (Levine sign) but if he can pinpoint with aid of a finger the exact site of pain (pointing sign) then it is likely to be local musculoskeletal pain.

☐ Patient is having acute onset of chest pain left side with breathlessness, how will you differentiate it from left sided pneumothorax and from left side pulmonary artery embolism?
Answer: In myocardial infarct, usually the pain and breathlessness increases gradually and is never "maximum" at the outset where as the pneumothorax and pulmonary embolism patient has an instantaneous onset of chest pain and breathlessness, which is very severe right from the beginning. Moreover, in pulmonary embolism (massive) patient can go into shock immediately, cardiogenic shock and LV failure takes time to develop and is usually gradual.

☐ How can you tell only by history whether the breathlessness is cardiac or respiratory in origin?
Answer: Besides of course the history of cardiac disease (infarct, vavular defects, hypertension, etc.) or respiratory disease (episodic bronchial asthma, chronic smoker's bronchitis, pulmonary tuberculosis.), cough usually precedes breathlessness in respiratory diseases, is associated with thick tenacious sputum (in contrast to pink frothy sputum of cardiac asthma) paroxysmal nocturnal dyspnea is more a feature of cardiac asthma; however even respiratory disease patients feel less breathless in sitting position due to improved vital capacity as intra-abdominal viscera move away from diaphragm. Patient typically holding the railing of bed to make use of accessory muscles of respiration is a sign of respiratory cause for breathlessness. Rhonchi or whistling musical sounds during respiratory efforts (wheeze) though considered a sign for bronchial asthma/

bronchitis may sometimes to be present as a result of reflex bronchospasm in LVF so be aware of the axiom "all that wheezes is not asthma" just as "all that glitters is not gold".

☐ Palpitations are mostly cardiac or noncardiac in origin. Which patient is more likely to complain of palpitations, a case of AF or frequent ventricular ectopic? Which beat is felt by patient with ventricular extra systole?
Answer: Mostly palpitations are noncardiac in origin especially in young persons with anxiety, neurocirculatory asthenia. Many times the palpitations are due to benign ectopics even in healthy individuals. A case of frequent PVCs is more likely to complain of palpitations rather than patient with chronic atrial fibrillation who gets "used" to his/her heart beats. The beat which is 'extra' is usually not felt by patient but the beat following the extra systolic, the post-extra-systolic beat is felt as heart contracts more powerfully following increased filling during the compensatory pause following ventricular extra systole.

☐ Why the NYHA grading of disability is not very satisfactory way of grading?
Answer: It is very subjective for enquiry Ordinary physical activity may vary from person to person.

For a marathon runner, running more than 20 miles may be "ordinary physical activity" but for a busy businessman walking from his car to the lift and from lift to his car back again may be "ordinary physical activity" and obviously class III (symptoms on less than ordinary physical activity) may be totally different in the two individuals. Moreover, we cannot tell the severity of illness just by this grading, patient may have serious heart illness (severe CAD) with just mild symptoms and vice versa. Sometimes the patient of mitral stenosis who was class II, overnight becomes class IV (symptomatic at rest) because of onset of atrial fibrillation, certainly the mitral valve cannot become critically narrow overnight so we cannot correlate severity of illness with symptoms.

☐ What is "angina inversus"?
Answer: When pain of angina starts from it little finger and radiates towards center of chest.

☐ What is "angina decubitus"
Answer: Angina in lying down position likely to be due to increased myocardial oxygen consumption due to increase venous return.

☐ How will the patient of dextrocardia with angina present to you?
Answer: He will complain of right sided chest pain with radiation to right arm (inner side).

■ PHYSICAL EXAMINATION

Pulse

☐ What is the purpose of three fingers for feeling radial artery in the wrist?
Answer: Proximal finger is used to gradually increase the pressure on the artery to guess the pressure required to make artery impalpable by the middle finger. It gives rough estimate of pulse pressure and compressibility of the artery. Middle finger is used to assess rate, rhythm, volume, character and condition of vessel wall. To assess condition of vessel wall, the proximal finger obliterates the radial artery, middle finger squeezes the flow distally to make it empty and the distal finger then compresses the radial artery to prevent its refilling by ulnar artery through palmer arch.

☐ Which is the best artery to look for Bisferiens pulse ?
Answer: Carotid artery may show it but better felt in peripheral arteries.

☐ Usually the post extrasystolic pulse is felt more powerfully because of its increased volume, in which condition post-extrasystolic beat is weaker?
Answer: In HOCM—Hypertrophic obstructive cardliomyopathy.

In this condition the increased force of contraction of post-extrasystolic beat increases the dynamic obstruction of the outflow tract making the pulse weak (Brockenbrough's sign).

- Can we get raised JVP in conditions associated with LVH/LVF ?

  Answer: Yes due to bulging of IVS into the RV side (Bernheim sign).

- Normally, JVP falls during inspiration. In which condition it increases?

  Answer: In constrictive Pericarditis – as the increased venous return during inspiration cannot be accommodated in RV, RA due to pericardial constriction (Kussmaul's sign).

- What is the logic behind measuring JVP after propping up patient at 45º, from the horizontal level? Will the "jugular venous pressure" be different in different postures?

  Answer: The most logical reason is that at 45º most of the persons with normal Jugular venous pressure will have no perceptible pulsations above the level of clavicle or at the most will have up to 3 cm above the horizontal level at sternal angle. Even in many of patients with CCF the upper level of internal jugular venous pulsations can be seen in the neck. It is measurable at 45º in majority of persons. Many persons will have JVP below clavicle in sitting position and above angle of jaw in lying down hence not measurable. jugular venous pressure and description of various waves can be seen better. Moreover if JVP is not raised hepato jugular reflux can be elicited better in 45 º positions.

  As for as actual measurement is concerned, "jugular venous pressure" will remain almost the same at different angles.

- In which condition JVP is raised but has no pulsations?

  Answer: In superior mediastinal obstruction.

- As the internal jugular vein is deep and due to thick skin/fascia, it may not be visible, how can you make the venous pulsation more easily visible ?

Answer: By "Shadow effect", with the aid of a sharp focus torch throw a shadow of the edge of a paper or scale in the superficial skin on anatomical line of internal jugular vein (from between two heads of sternocleidomastoid to angle of mandible). Shadow will be seen to be moving like undulations of a straight-line shadow and hence you can see the upper level of pulsations. Now draw a horizontal plane at this level with aid of a thin paper or scale, draw another horizontal plane at the level of sternal angle. Both planes should be parallel to the ground and hence parallel to each other. Measure the vertical distance between the two planes. Normally it should be up to 3 cm, add 5 cm. to it as center of right atrium is 5 cm deep to the sternal angle so nomal JVP is 8 cm of water or blood (as the manometric tube here is internal jugular vein).

- How are the 'a' waves in atrial fibrillation?

  Answer: 'A' wave are absent in AF as there is no effective atrial contractions.

- From which part of chest should you start looking for and palpating for apex beat.

  Answer: Always start from posterior auxiliary line otherwise, you may miss grossly enlarged heart.

- What is the character of normal apex beat and in mitral stenosis?

  Answer: Normal apex beat character is described as "tapping" (touches your finger and goes without lifting it). In mitral stenosis also, description is same tapping but mechanism is different here it is considered to be due to palpable first heart found and RVH.

- What is the diagnostic and unambiguous physical sign of pericardial effusion?

  Answer: If you can demonstrate by percussion that cardiac dullness is extending beyond the apex beat then it has to be pericardial effusion.... !

- In which condition you can get "double apex beat" in one heartbeat.

Answer: HOCM (hypertrophic cardiomyopathy,) in LV apical aneurysm you can get "bifid apex beat".

- How can you make a mild parasternal heave more visible?

  Answer: By keeping a pencil horizontally on left parasternal area and seeing the movements of this pencil by sitting with eyes at level of this horizontal pencil and seeing tangentially against a contrast background.

- Normally with RVH, you get a positive thrust in the parasternal area with upward movement of the chest wall in supine position, can you get an inward or downward movement of chest wall in presence of RVH.

  Answer: Yes, in organic TR (No PAH) during RV contraction, there is systolic collapse/downward movement of the chest wall, At this time apex beat is moving up. So you get what is called "Sea saw movement" of the chest wall, apex beat area moving up and parasternal area going down (seen in organic tricuspid regurgitation TR).

- When actually there is reduction in LV volume during systole why do you get outward movement of the apex beat in systole?

  Answer: It is because the left ventricle contracts during systole just like you wearing a wet towel, it rotates around longitudinal axis since LV is firmly anchored at level of base of heart due to great vessels, the apex rotates and strikes against the chest wall....!

- How much extra fluid must be accumulated in an adult before we get pitting edema in the legs ?

  Answer: Approximately ten liters, hence an early sign of CCF is gain in weight (One liter equals approx one kg.)

- Usually patient is cold and clammy in states of shock, tell a condition where it is not so?

  Answer: In septicemia shock (warm shock).

- Can you have enlarged and tender liver in CCF with no pedal edema and normal JVP?

  Answer: Yes, if the patient has been treated especially with diuretics, due to its spongy nature liver takes a long time to regress to its smaller size...!

- What is the earliest physical sign of CCF ?

  Answer: Hepatojugular reflux/gain in weight.

- Cyanosis is often associated with breath lessness, tell me some conditions in which despite intense cyanosis patient is not breathless...!

  Answer:
  a. Cyanosis due to methemoglobinemia.
  b. Differential cyanosis PDA with reversal of shunt—Deoxygenated blood goes to lower limbs.

- In which situation "sinus arrhythmia" is absent? Otherwise, it is nomal!

  Answer:
  1. In conditions associated with autonomic neuropathy (eg diabetic).
  2. Full atropinization.
  3. Transplanted heart.
  4. Patient on pacemaker.

- Normally right heart events are accentuated with inspiration exception being ?

  Answer: Pulmonary ejection click.

- Why the murmur of mitral regurgitation is radiated widely to axilla but murmur of mitral stenosis is "localized at apex with no radiation ?

  Answer: Radiation of murmur depends on direction of the jet of blood flow, which is producing the murmur.

  The regurgitant jet in MR is going from LV to LA (most posterior chamber of the heart) hence murmur is radiated to axilla.

  In MS, the blood flow producing the diastolic murmur is from LA to LV apex, since the LV apex is corresponding to apex beat the murmur cannot radiate anywhere else and is localized to apex.

- Usually all the murmurs decrease in standing position except two—which are these two conditions?

  Answer: HOCM and MVP show increase in systolic murmurs with standing (due to reduced LV volume).

- How will you differentiate between mid-diastolic murmur of MS and mid diastolic murmur heard at apex in severe AR (Austin flint murmur).

Answer: Absence of thrill, absence of opening snap and absence of loud first heart sound are seen in distinguishing features of Austin flint murmur.

- How will you differentiate between Carey Combs murmur (in rheumatic carditis) and diastolic murmur of established organic MS?
  Answer: Cary Combs murmur is not associated with thrill, first heart sound is soft and there is no opening snap.

- What is "Occult MS" ?
  Answer: Physical signs especially auscultatory signs of MS may be absent at times in severe MS (even needing urgent surgery or BMV).

- Physical signs of ventricular fibrillation are same as "death" unconsciousness no respiration, no pulse, no BP, no heart sounds but what is the difference?
  Answer: The most important basic difference is that Ventricular fibrillation is reversible. In more than 95% of patients with primary ventricular fibrillation the rhythm converts to sinus rhythm by properly timed (within 1–2 minutes) DC shock. Most of these persons leave the hospital alive.

- If you are posted as a medical officer somewhere in rural areas of south India and a middle-aged man is brought to you with severe bradycardia likely to be complete heart block. History is of trying to commit suicide by ingesting some poison. What will you suspect and do?
  Answer: Eating "Kaner Seeds" is a common mode of committing suicide. It causes severe bradycardia and CHB. Pulse, cannon waves (irregular), variable intensity of S is common clinical diagnostic features. Treatment is to tide over period by temporary pacing. (Kaner is a tree with milk like juice in stem leaves.)

- What is pseudohypertension?
  Answer: It is a condition where brachial arteries have become thickened calcific due to atherosclerotic process and become increasingly stiff and non-compressible and increased pressure needed in sphygmo manometer cuff to obliterate pulsations. Intra arterial recording may not be high.

- What is the full form of ECG? Electrocardiogram/Electrocardiograph?
  Answer: The tracing that you read is electrocardiogram (not graph as expected by many) and the machine is electrocardiograph machine.

Some teasers – I am not giving answer here – dig out, explore and find otherwise 'e-mail' the author for answers:

1. ECG typically shows "low voltage" in pericardial effusion. Fluid is a good conductor of electricity then why low voltage?
2. What is reversed pulse paradoxus? In which condition you get it?
3. In which condition VT may be induced by telephone call bell ring early in the morning?
4. What are the physical signs including cardiac auscultation in case with 'Transplanted heart'?

   This condition is called occult MS, this is because of severe PAH leading to poor cardiac output, poor LA filling and reduced flow through narrow MV orifice hence turbulence is less and murmur may not be heard. Opening snap may not be audible as OS may be too close to S_2 to be heard.

- What is Tropical MS?
  Answer: Seen is India and Asian developing countries tempo of disease is fast, calcification more and earlier, Af is earlier.

- We commonly describe a typical murmur of mitral stenosis as "mid-diastolic rumble". What do you understand by the term "Rumble".
  Answer: Rumble literally means a sound like "thunder of distant clouds" – a typical low-pitched series of sounds which is heard just as we hear murmur of MS.

- We often describe typical brachial and radial pulse of severe aortic regurgitation as "Water hammer pulse". What is "Water hammer"?
  Answer: Water hammer was the name given to a Japanese toy enjoyed by children. It is a hollow sealed glass cubicle. Half of cubicle is vacuum and the other half is having water. Child tilts the cubical upside down and water rushes to the vacuum area and a "thud" is felt. Now the child reverses the direction and again 'thud' is felt. Same feeling we get over brachial artery in AR.

- How can you mimic murmur of aortic regurgitation-one of the difficult murmurs to be recognized clinically?
  Answer: Hold your folded palm in front of your open mouth and forcibly perform expiration into the hollow of hands the sound heard typically resembles AR murmur.

- Pericarditis is typically very painful. Can you tell a variety of pericarditis which is painless? And why it is painless?
  Answer: Uremic pericarditis. Only the inferior part of pericardium is sensitive to pain. Most of cases of pericarditis are infective and the pain is mostly due to associated infection and inflammation of contiguous pleura. Uremic pericarditis being non infectious may not-involve the pleura and hence may be painless.

- If God gives you a choice, either you suffer from mitral slenosis or from aortic regurgitation or aortic stenosis, what will you chose and why?
  Answer: Of course, nobody will like to chose any of these but if it is God's wish then one should chose aortic valve disease. Reason being that patients with M.S. become symptomatic very early with breathlessness, because increased LA pressure is directly transmitted to pulmonary veins and capillaries leading to increased pulmonary edema. Moreover, MS patients have episodes of thromboembolisms more often.

- In severe aortic stenosis (valvular) patient has history of syncope after exertion and not during exertion – why?
  Answer: During exertion, patient has more venous return which can compensate for increased skeletal muscle blood needs (fulfilled by skeletal muscle vessel dilation). After exertion is over the skeletal muscle blood vessels continue to be in dilated state for some time but venous return decreases hence cerebral blood flow suffers as the blood flows preferentially to skeletal muscles at the expense of brain.

- If in a case with unconsciousness and generalized convulsions, pulse is found to be below 40/min. what will you suspect?
  Answer: We should suspect "stokes Adam's attack" due to complete heart block and get it confirmed by ECG.

- What are the physical signs of complete heart block (acquired) ?
  Answer: Slow pulse and heart rate (usually less than 40/min.) high pulse pressures, irregular cannon waves in JVP, variable intensity of first heart sound.

- If a young person complains of chest pain that in relieved by exertion- what will be your diagnosis?
  Answer: Most likely this is a functional problem, psychosomatic in nature, neurocirculataory asthenia. It usually rules out organic cause.

Index

Herpes zoster 9
Hill's sign 116
His bundle 160
Homans sign 33
Horner's syndrome 26*f*
Hydrothorax 74
Hypercholesterolemia, familial 3
Hyperlipidemia 3
Hypertension 3, 26, 26*f*, 154
    clinical features of 59
    in pregnancy 153, 154
    malignant 66
    pulmonary 83, 88, 98, 141
Hyperthyroidism 27*f*
Hypotension 148
    causes of 148

I

Icterus 22*f*
Idiopathic cardiomyopathy 129
Idiopathic myocarditis 129
Incompetence, pulmonary 99, 117
Infarction, pulmonary 100
Infective endocarditis 126

J

Janeway's lesion 124
Jockman's dictum 124
Jugular pulse 74
Jugular vein, examination of 31*f*
Jugular venous pressure, measurement of 30*f*

K

Keith-Wagener classification 64
Kidney disease 3
Koilonychia 25*f*
Kussmaul's sign 29, 138

L

Liver engorgement 73
Loeffler's syndrome 129
Lung disease 76, 143, 145, 150

M

Marfan's syndrome 3, 79
Mitral incompetence 94, 102, 104
    clinical findings of 103
Mitral stenosis 95, 156, 164
Mitral valve disease 94
    causes of 95
    classification of 94
Mitral valve prolapse 103
    clinical findings of 103
Mitral valvotomy 119
Mixed mitral stenosis and incompetence
        94, 100
Murmurs 48, 74
    continuous 48
    delayed 47
    diastolic 47, 97
    ejection 46
    pansystolic 46
    presystolic 47
    systolic 46, 135
Musset's sign 116
Myocardial disease 129, 130
Myocardial infarction 53
    pain of 8
Myocarditis 129, 130
Myxedema 157
    heart 157

N

Nausea 53
Neurofibromatosis 26, 26*f*
Nocturia 12

O

Obstruction cardiomyopathy, hypertrophic
        111, 134
Opening snap 97
Orthopnea 70
Osler's nodes 124
Ostium primum defects 79

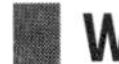 **W**

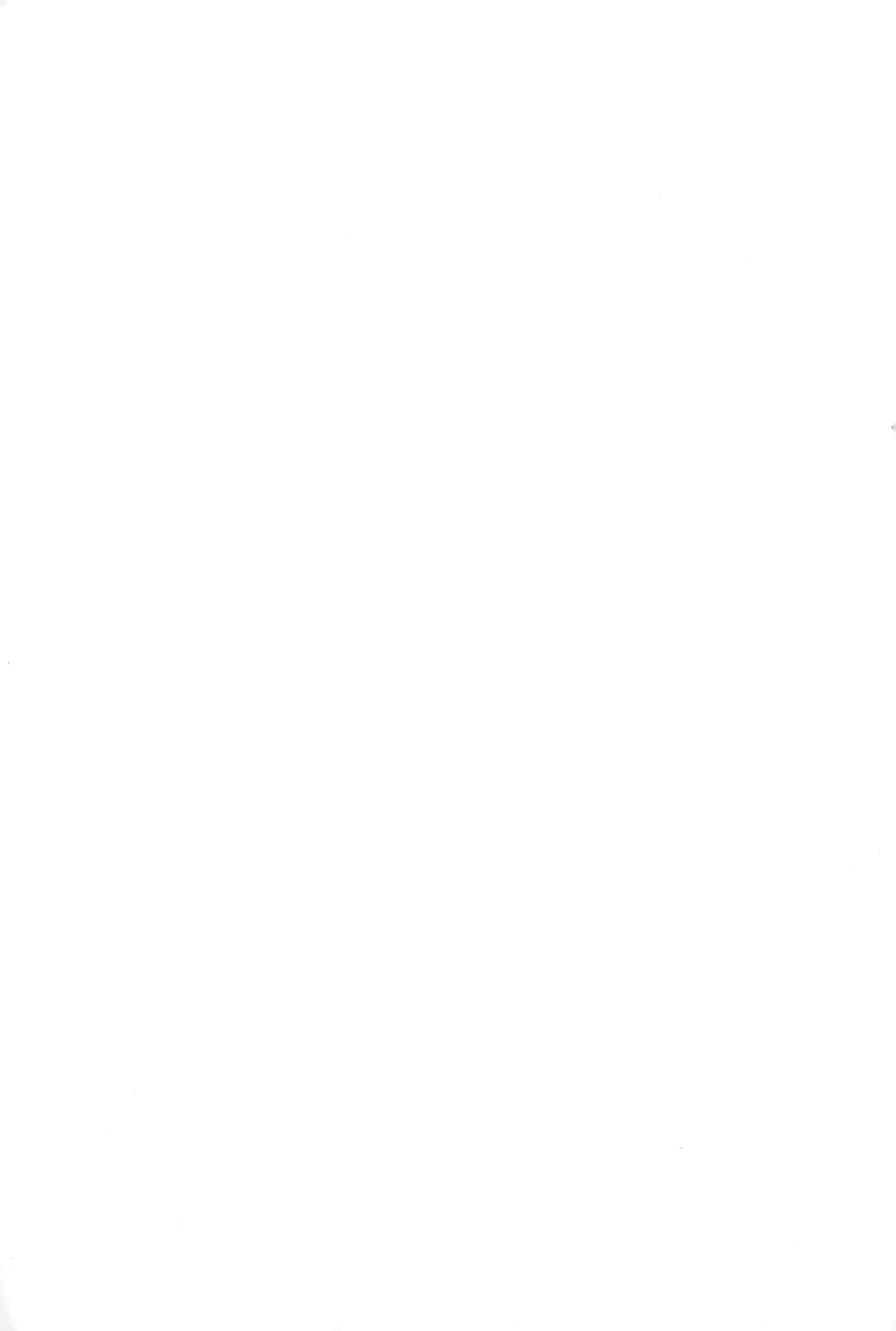